T0231269

Psychosocial Approaches to Deeply Disturbed Persons

Peter R. Breggin
E. Mark Stern
Editors

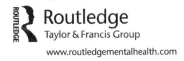

Routledge
Taylor & Francis Group

www.routledgementalhealth.com

Transferred to digital printing 2010 by Routledge

Routledge
Taylor and Francis Group
270 Madison Avenue
New York, NY 10016

Routledge
Taylor and Francis Group
2 Park Square
Milton Park, Abingdon
Oxon OX14 4RN

Psychosocial Approaches to Deeply Disturbed Persons has also been published as *The Psychotherapy Patient*, Volume 9, Numbers 3/4 1996.

The development, preparation, and publication of this work has been undertaken with great care. However, the publisher, employees, editors, and agents of The Haworth Press and all imprints of The Haworth Press, Inc., including The Haworth Medical Press and Pharmaceutical Products Press, are not responsible for any errors contained herein or for consequences that may ensue from use of materials or information contained in this work. Opinions expressed by the author(s) are not necessarily those of The Haworth Press, Inc.

The Haworth Press, Inc., 10 Alice Street, Binghamton, NY 13904-1580 USA

Library of Congress Cataloging-in-Publication Data

Psychosocial approaches to deeply disturbed persons / Peter R. Breggin, E. Mark Stern, editors.
    p. cm.
    Includes bibliographical references.
    ISBN 1-56024-841-6
    1. Schizophrenia. 2. Schizophrenia–Treatment. 3. Schizophrenics–Rehabilitation. I. Breggin, Peter Roger, 1936- II. Stern, E. Mark, 1929- .
    RC514.P71886 1996
    616.89′82–dc20   96-12677
                                               CIP

Psychosocial Approaches to Deeply Disturbed Persons

CONTENTS

ABOUT THE EDITORS

Peter R. Breggin, MD, is a psychiatrist in private practice in Bethesda, Maryland, and the founder of the Center for the Study of Psychiatry and Psychology. He is also Faculty Associate, Department of Counseling and Human Services, The Johns Hopkins University.

Dr. Breggin is the author of many books and articles, most recently *Toxic Psychiatry* (1991), *Beyond Conflict* (1992), and with Ginger Ross Breggin, *Talking Back to Prozac* (1994) and *The War Against Children* (1994), all published by St. Martin's Press. He has two forthcoming books, *The Heart of Being Helpful* and *Brain-Disabling Treatments in Psychiatry*, both scheduled for 1997 from Springer Publishing Company.

E. Mark Stern, EdD, is Professor Emeritus in the Graduate Faculty of Arts and Sciences, Iona College, New Rochelle, New York. A Diplomate in Clinical Psychology of the American Board of Professional Psychology and a Fellow of the American Psychological Association, the American Psychological Society, and the Academy of Clinical Psychology, Dr. Stern has been President of the Divisions of Humanistic Psychology and Psychology of Religion, APA. He is in private practice of psychotherapy with offices at 215 East Eleventh Street, New York, NY 10003.

Introduction:
Spearheading a Transformation

Peter R. Breggin

In recent years, pharmacology and psychiatric hospitalization have become the standard for most professionals when "treating schizophrenia." Meanwhile, a body of research and practical experience has been evolving that supports innovative psychosocial interventions as less hazardous and more effective. As psychiatry goes through still another historical cycle in the conflict between psychosocial and biological approaches, we may be on the verge of a renewed emphasis on human service interventions. This book hopes to spearhead such a transformation by reviewing current research, theory and practice based on the psychosocial model.

PERSONS AS AGENTS AND BEINGS

How we view human beings in general is fundamental to the controversy over how to conceptualize and approach deeply disturbed, seem-

---

Author Note: The title of the book, *Psychosocial Approaches to Deeply Disturbed Persons*, reflects its orientation. Because the term *treatment* tends to encourage a biopsychiatric or medical model, I have chosen the term *approach* as an alternative. How to approach or "come near to" the labeled patient is often critical. Similarly, the term *schizophrenic* narrows the scope of professional roles and viewpoints. Therefore the book title addresses *deeply disturbed people*—those who are profoundly troubled and anguished, and who often receive severe psychiatric labels, such as schizophrenia. Because of the wide variety of viewpoints represented by the contributors and because of the need to communicate in a commonly accepted language, the terms *treatment* and *schizophrenia* will nonetheless recur throughout the chapters.

[Haworth co-indexing entry note]: "Introduction: Spearheading a Transformation." Breggin, Peter R. Co-published simultaneously in *The Psychotherapy Patient* (The Haworth Press, Inc.) Vol. 9, No. 3/4, 1996, pp. 1-7; and: *Psychosocial Approaches to Deeply Disturbed Persons* (eds: Peter R. Breggin, and E. Mark Stern) The Haworth Press, Inc., 1996, pp. 1-7. Single or multiple copies of this article are available from The Haworth Document Delivery Service [1-800-342-9678, 9:00 a.m. - 5:00 p.m. (EST)].

ingly irrational people. I believe that all individuals should be viewed as agents and beings (Breggin, 1991, 1992, 1997).

People as *agents* are active forces in their own lives. In philosophical terms, they have autonomy and are capable of self-determination. Free will may have its limitations, including those imposed by genetics and biology, but the effective exercise of free will is critical to recovery and to successful living. Because human beings must exercise free will in order to survive and to prosper, they need a maximum of personal freedom. Thus the principle of liberty becomes crucial to human progress on both the personal and political level (Breggin, 1992). Approaches to deeply disturbed human beings should as much as possible respect their autonomy, independence, and freedom. They should seek to *increase* rather than to limit their liberty.

People as *beings* not only have agency or the ability to take actions, more specifically they are capable of generating values, including love. They can offer love and they can accept it. Love is an active, positive attitude toward others, a treasuring of others that is reverent, caring, and empathic. The capacity to share love is central to recovery and to continued personal growth (Breggin, 1997).

The principles of liberty and love–and relationships based on them–empower individuals, enabling them to overcome trauma stress, and to live their fullest potential. On the one hand, empowerment is healing. It soothes pain and anguish. On the other, it is strengthening–it supports the individual's pursuit of his or her own chosen values and ideals.

Persons are influenced and constrained by their bodies, and they require their bodies in order to function; but they exist as well on a level that is variously called psychological, psychosocial, existential, or psychospiritual. They *generate* thoughts and feelings, they *create* values and meanings, they *choose* courses of actions, and they *relate* to other beings–influencing them and in turn being influenced by them. That is, they are both agents and beings.

Anguished, self-defeating responses to life, from anxiety and despair to madness, are learned through hurtful interactions with ourselves, other people, and life. Often these responses can be understood as "psychospiritual overwhelm" (Breggin, 1991). In a somewhat simplified manner, I have described the origin of this helplessness in the basic stress paradigm of hurt, fear and helplessness (Breggin, 1992, pp. 103-104; 1997). The individual becomes helpless in the face of seeming personal devastation from internal and external threats. Healing requires overcoming helplessness through self-understanding, rational thought processes, loving attitudes, positive values and ideals, effective choices and actions, and loving relationships.

PERSONS AS OBJECTS OR BIOCHEMICAL DEVICES

The "scientific" or scientistic approach takes a starkly contrasting attitude toward those who suffer mental disturbances and anguish, especially those who end up with psychotic labels (e.g., schizophrenia, major depression and manic-depressive disorder).[1] In the extreme, the person is seen as a reactive object or biological mechanism. He or she becomes an "it" devoid of the capacity to generate thoughts or feelings, to create values or meanings, to choose courses of action, or to influence and be influenced by others. Or if the person is granted these human capacities, the capacities are seen as irrelevant to the processes involved in "mental illness" and "treatment" (Breggin and Breggin, 1994a & b).

In previous decades, the scientistic approach in psychiatry included both a biological and an environmental wing. The individual's behavior was seen as determined by either biological variables or environmental ones; but either way, the principles of cause and effect applied. In more recent times, environmental determinism has lost its verge and been largely replaced by genetic and biochemical determinism. Environment has come to play almost no role in the thinking of many modern psychiatrists, especially in regard to the "causation" of severe "mental illnesses," such as major depression, manic-depressive disorder, and schizophrenia (reviewed in Breggin, 1991).

More "balanced" or "eclectic" psychiatric perspectives tend to include both genetic predispositions and environmental influences. These are usually found in textbooks of psychiatry. In actual practice, however, most current theories and textbooks tend to emphasize genetic and biochemical factors and to encourage physical treatments. Even while giving passing mention to psychosocial theories and practices, these theories and textbooks display skepticism toward them. They devote no attention to psychospiritual issues, such as love.

CONTRASTING THERAPEUTIC APPROACHES

If we approach the human as a being, then our task is to understand and to empower. Understanding involves intuition, empathy and love. Empowerment involves self-understanding, moral encouragement through a caring relationship, and guidance toward more effective, autonomous and loving principles of living. It may also involve direct assistance in negotiating life's stresses, for example, by helping the individual become more effective in utilizing community resources or by including his or her family in the therapy.

If we approach the human "scientifically" or "objectively," then the tendency is to diagnose and to control, to impose our own abstract and potentially oppressive category upon the person, and to manipulate the outcome. Physical interventions, such as drugs and enforced confinement in a mental hospital, become the preferred tools (Breggin and Breggin, 1994a & b).

Often the patient feels *mis*understood, rather than understood; *dis*empowered rather than empowered. These approaches seem to empower the doctor far more than the patient.

The biopsychiatric approach can easily reinforce the patient's worst feelings and attitudes. The patient already feels helpless—at the mercy of forces beyond his or her control. The patient often feels like an object or thing that can do nothing more than react helplessly to internal and external threats. In the extreme, the individual suffers from delusions and hallucinations about being influenced and manipulated by imaginary others and outside unknown forces. Often the patient feels "mentally defective."

Unfortunately, the biopsychiatrist's approach will encourage the patient's self-destructive attitudes by further encouraging the patient to think and act like a helpless victim of overwhelming forces, namely, genetic and biochemical abnormalities. The doctor then "takes over" and prescribes physical agents that are supposed to counteract the genetic and biochemical influences. This further reinforces the patient's self-destructive helplessness.

The patient can easily become a passive battlefield between two warring parties—the forces of his or her own alleged biological abnormalities, and the forces of biopsychiatry in the form of drugs and electroshock. Whatever the seeming outcome, the patient's worst view of life is reconfirmed—that he or she is a passive victim of forces beyond personal understanding and control.

In an especially tragic irony, the biopsychiatrist frequently renders the patient *more helpless* by means of brain-disabling treatments and involuntary hospitalization (Breggin, 1991; Breggin & Breggin, 1994a & b). The patient—whose problems are driven by overwhelming feelings of helplessness—is further overwhelmed by coercive therapy and brain dysfunction.

PHILOSOPHY AND SCIENCE

There are, of course, not only philosophical considerations but scientific ones. To a great extent both the public and mental health profession has accepted the claim that so-called schizophrenia is a genetic and biochemical disease, and that drugs, electroshock, and mental hospitals are effective, humane approaches to severe human suffering. The public, the media and much of the profession mistakenly believe that the biopsychiatrists have a corner on the scientific market.

I have critiqued this "science" in *Toxic Psychiatry: Why Therapy, Empathy, and Love Must Replace the Drugs, Electroshock and Biochemical Theories of the 'New Psychiatry'* (1991), as well as in a variety of other professional publications (Breggin, 1979, 1983; Breggin and Breggin, 1994a & b). Karon and Whitaker will continue that analysis in their chapter in this book. I will not try to duplicate or to summarize the arguments and evidence already offered in rebuttal, except to say that biopsychiatric claims are largely without foundation. There is no convincing evidence to support genetic and biochemical theories or the physical interventions so highly touted by contemporary biopsychiatry. Most available scientific evidence instead undermines biopsychiatric theory and practice.

Scientific research does have a place in the helping professions, for example, in testing theories and more practically in the evaluation of "outcomes." But any attempt to evaluate the results of a therapeutic approach will reflect the researchers' underlying values, often expressed in the variables which are selected for evaluation. For example, studies that demonstrate the effectiveness of drugs for depression typically focus on symptom relief, such as weight gain or reduced insomnia. These studies merely reconfirm the well-known fact that many drugs, including tricyclic antidepressants, can physically stimulate appetite and cause sedation. On the other hand, research that demonstrates the efficacy of psychotherapy tends to focus on subjective changes in the patient's feelings and on actual changes in lifestyle or the conduct of life (Fisher and Greenberg, 1989). Psychotherapy is more effective than medication when these criteria are used.

Psychosocial research should place much more emphasis on the patient's personal or subjective response to "treatment." In biopsychiatry, patients who are medicated or shocked are typically labeled "improved" when they conform to hospital demands or receive discharge from the hospital. But the patients themselves often feel badly drugged, befuddled, or coerced. Often they actively resist the supposedly beneficial treatment by secretly spitting out their pills or by pleading for an end to shock treatment. Increased discharge rates often reflect the desire to escape from escalating treatment with drugs or shock (Breggin, 1979, 1983, 1991).

Unfortunately, it is difficult to find research that takes into account the patient or client's personal, subjective response, or that examines beneficial changes in lifestyle. We end up trying to infer benefits from other variables, such as length or frequency of hospitalization, that bear little relationship to overall improvement in mood, attitudes or lifestyle.

A CONFLICT RESOLUTION MODEL

People who come to the attention of mental health professionals are in conflict. Their conflicts may be internal, and characterized by guilt, shame, anxiety, numbing and anger. Or they may be external or "behavioral," involving others in their lives and society. The more severely "ill" they seem, the more they are embroiled in severe conflict–within themselves and with others, often including active strife with mental health professionals who try to treat.

Conflict resolution based on respect for the principles of liberty and love provides an effective contemporary model for the mental health profession. It addresses the basic needs of each individual involved in the conflict and seeks to increase their satisfaction (Breggin, 1992, 1997). It calls for creating a safe space for the individual in which coercive power is replaced by reason, love, and mutual attempts to satisfy the basic needs of those involved in the conflict.

Unfortunately, much of the mental health profession relies on the medical model which seeks to identify one member of the conflict as the "cause of it all" and further seeks to locate the "cause" within the labeled individual's genetic and biochemical vulnerability. In the process it frequently revictimizes one of the victims of the conflict, while it ignores the larger psychological, familial, social and political context of the conflict. Often it utilizes coercive power in the form of brain-disabling treatments and involuntary hospitalization.

Deeply disturbed people should be viewed as persons struggling to survive and to grow–as persons in conflict with themselves and with other people. Healing comes through a combination of self-development and beneficial relationships with others. It is maximized when people are treated as agents and beings, according to the ideals of liberty and love.

NOTE

1. Scientism is the misapplication of the principles of the physical sciences to understanding human mental life and conduct. It emphasizes simple-minded cause and effect reactivity at the expense of volition and subjectively-chosen values.

REFERENCES

Breggin, P. R. (1979). *Electroshock: Its brain-disabling effects.* New York: Springer Publishing Company.

Breggin, P. R. (1983). *Psychiatric drugs: Hazards to the brain.* New York: Springer.

Breggin, P. R. (1991). *Toxic psychiatry: Why therapy, empathy and love must replace the drugs, electroshock and biochemical theories of the 'new psychiatry'.* New York: St. Martin's Press.

Breggin, P. R. (1992). *Beyond conflict: From self-help and psychotherapy to peacemaking.* New York: St. Martin's Press.

Breggin, P. R. & Breggin, G. (1994a). *Talking back to Prozac: What doctors aren't telling you about today's most controversial drug.* New York: St. Martin's Press.

Breggin, P. R., & Breggin, G. (1994b). *The war against children: The government's intrusion into schools, families and communities in search of a medical "cure" for violence.* New York: St. Martin's Press.

Breggin, P. R. (1997, in press) *The heart of being helpful.* New York: Springer Publishing Company.

Fisher, S., & Greenberg, R. (1989). *The limits of biological treatments for psychological distress: Comparisons with psychotherapy and placebo.* Hillsdale, New Jersey: Lawrence Erlbaum.

Schizophrenic Experience:
A Humanistic Perspective

E. Mark Stern

SUMMARY. Schizophrenic consciousness is an alternative view of life, common to the human predicament as a means of psychic endurance. Psychosis diffuses identity. In so doing, the crazymaking person tends to be locked into symbiosis, cementing this closure through automatically yielding to the demands of others via the passageway of depersonalizing depression and anxiety. *[Article copies available from The Haworth Document Delivery Service: 1-800-342-9678.]*

ALTERNATIVE REALITIES

In the 1902 Gifford Lectures, delivered at the University of Edinburgh, William James (1958) expressed concern that alternative "forms of (human) consciousness (tend to be) disregarded." Paying serious attention to experiential variations of conscious awareness is, in Jamesian terms, an essential inquiry, without which psychology stands in danger of promoting " . . . a premature closing of our accounts with reality" (p. 298). Schizophrenic consciousness acts as an alternative to a world filled with intracultural contradictions.

Each era confers meaning on the problems of being in the world. In our time, as in others, confusing cultural sentiments abound. Some of the fallout from these social bewilderments involves alternative sensibilities. Among these alternative modes of being, schizophrenia reflects the condition of a person whose relations to the current demands of sanity have

[Haworth co-indexing entry note]: "Schizophrenic Experience: A Humanistic Perspective." Stern, E. Mark. Co-published simultaneously in *The Psychotherapy Patient* (The Haworth Press, Inc.) Vol. 9, No. 3/4, 1996, pp. 9-21; and: *Psychosocial Approaches to Deeply Disturbed Persons* (eds: Peter R. Breggin, and E. Mark Stern) The Haworth Press, Inc., 1996, pp. 9-21. Single or multiple copies of this article are available from The Haworth Document Delivery Service [1-800-342-9678, 9:00 a.m. - 5:00 p.m. (EST)].

become broken (May, 1983). Nevertheless, the schizophrenic expresses this break by devoting his or her existence to the reversibilities of commonly accepted realities. In its haste to define and isolate models of disease driven behavior, society has demonstrated an increasing reliance on neuropsychiatric models (Torrey, 1995). Schizophrenics are widely regarded as diseased. Labeling schizophrenia as a sickness in wait of a cure well suits the dehumanizing signs of the times. The current emphasis on neuropsychiatric models further increases this society's dependence on differential diagnostic codes resulting in the inevitable growing use of biochemical, electroconvulsive and surgical "correctives."

SCHIZOPHRENIA AS A MODE OF BEING

Schizophrenia is a multi-axis combination of genetic, biochemical, psycho-social and developmental forces. Nonetheless, since social and technological conditions tend to determine the role deviant behaviors in any one time span, the schizophrenic phenomenon plays out its own contemporary existential theme. Even as an alienated mode of being, schizophrenia persists in redefining the current relationships of objects, space and time. Schizophrenic imagery speaks to relationships in its unique surreal language. As a dissident alternative to experience of "acceptable" relationships, schizophrenic associations are rarely static. Appreciated as a necessary agitator to other means of psychic endurance and survival, schizophrenic experience makes few distinctions between subjects and objects. Instead, schizophrenia connects with primordial linkages to primitive formats of language and perception. And while specific schizophrenic behaviors are more prominent in certain individuals, the broader population of non-psychotics may at times embody similar deviations and detachments. Dreams and hypnagogic states in the nonpsychotic, compare well to the visions of the schizophrenic.

DISENGAGEMENT AND CONVENTION

Labeled clinically as a serious thought disorder, schizophrenia is, in fact, a tousled scramble of estranged inventiveness and poetic cosmic speculations. Within schizophrenic consciousness, bizarre images reassess familiar conclusions. Contradiction, digression and mania knot themselves to the task of the schizophrenic's being in society, and this by his or her ultimately despairing of intrusive normative social demands. Schizophrenic disengagement from objective reality devolves personhood into a further disengagement from society even as the psychosis forges new links to alternative constructs. To be sure, schizophrenic challenges to normative reality are often accompanied by frenzies and violent ecstasies. But even in their extreme, these explosive expressions never relent in serving as a persistent and tenacious surreal view of life, ultimately affecting all boundary negotiations (Stern, 1986). Yet, even as schizophrenic images necessarily duel with conventional imagery, conventional neuropsychiatric approaches are characteristically charged with the task of conventionalizing schizophrenic behavior.

Affective States

The affective life of schizophrenics is interwoven with strands of depression. Such depressive imagery is not mere joylessness. Nevertheless, the value of all phenomena are determined by the views taken of them. Neuropsychiatry and behaviorally-oriented psychology have waged their respective battle cries against the sometimes necessary messages of depression. Paul Schilder (1952), a pioneer in the psychotherapy of schizophrenics, considers the process of being schizophrenic as a more primitive mode of existence. Schilder observed that the schizophrenic is not contented with such primitivism, and that the continuing search for newer adaptations and even "progressive tendencies" is his or her way to move into closer contact with the world. Schilder was cautious, if not pessimistic, regarding the ordinary therapeutic successes with schizophrenic individuals. It behooves contemporary institutional mental illness personnel to extinguish all affective irregularities. As a result it is not uncommon for a post-medicated depressive to insist that he or she lives on a flat horizon, malnourished of former feelings.

Boundaries between schizophrenia and mood disorders are often quite arbitrary. Delusions combine affective deprivation with compensating furies. Disturbances in expression are often incomplete attempts at coping with a combined sense of hopelessness and grandiosity. Impasses in being able to feel effective often appear beyond repair. Despite this seeming hopelessness, schizophrenic imagery can be challenging in its own right. In the face of deep pain and "distortion" a psychotherapy patient, intent more on the struggle than on the solution wrote:

> I know I'm better because I feel worse. . . . The more lost I become the clearer it gets. . . . There is no winning or losing, but I keep what I have. (Deinelt, 1979, p. 231)

Being able to weigh in such struggles distinguishes what is schizophrenic depression, and may be apparent in any generic notion of schizophrenia.

Psychotic Despair

Schizophrenic consciousness can compromise itself into airtight lethargy. Viable tomorrows have little room to exist. Depression, linked to psychotic experience, appears incapable of reckoning with time. Many schizophrenics despair over ever having been born. "It is not," wrote Paul Tillich (1957), "the experience of time as such which produces (such) despair; rather it is defeat in the resistance against time (p. 69)."

For the schizophrenic, time is the ultimate illusion. There is no distinction between life and death. Identity is diffused. In its stead, symbiotic unions abound:

> Renata came into therapy at her twin brother's request. They had just turned 35. He described her as "silly" and depressive. Their mother had recently died of complications following a cerebral aneurysm. The aneurysm had caused a profound paralysis of left side. Renata had nursed her mother throughout the paralysis. Like her mother, she too was, according to her brother, "given to strange moods." On the day of her mother's death, Renata developed a Bell's palsy which had resulted in a temporary paralysis of the left side of her face. She was reminded by her brother, who accompanied her to the first session, of how profoundly sad she'd been. He spoke of the "strong connection" which had always existed between mother and daughter. Renata, on the other hand, claimed that she felt no need to grieve since "I see her face so clearly every time I look into a mirror." Renata felt alive in her mother's deadness. She refused to use the electrical device which had been prescribed to stimulate the left side of her face. Any restoration of movement felt forbidding. Renata's paralysis anesthetized her being. Stimulation meant "coming apart"— the feared "parting" from her mother.

Anxiety

Anxiety in the schizophrenic signifies further psychic and physical extinction. In contrast to schizoid depression, anxiety is linked to the terror of being and belonging. Otto Rank (1929) incorporates anxiety lay to the hub of the birth process. It might equally be speculated that the presence of anxiety is rooted in the echoes of the Big Bang of creation: the format of all cosmic uncertainty (Gauquelin, 1967).

Anxiousness within schizophrenia fails to confine the terrors of being lost within the immensity of existence within any suitable control. Consider Pascal's (1961) words:

> Whoever shall thus consider himself will be frightened at himself, and observing himself suspended in the mass of matter allotted to him by nature, between these two abysses of infinity and nothingness, will tremble at the sight of these wonders. (p. 47)

Fretfulness and apprehensiveness team together to delimit boundaries of personal reality. For the schizophrenic, anxiety is agoraphobic. This imprisonment fails to provide safety, leaving only a pervasive surrealism which, while appearing to be exotic, actually escalates into further disablement (Searles, 1961).

HARVEY: SEEING IT ALL

Harvey lived in a recurring dream. Day-to-day realities were sapped at their foundations. Images would toss and turn between worry, horselaughs and tears. Compulsions were indistinguishable from terrors. Harvey was in total collapse. Fleeting ruminations randomly scanned seemingly unrelated contexts. Time and body parts had become mere tracings of movement. Harvey's torments were unremitting. He fretted about his head being ripped into shreds. The idea of suicide was all that remained. Despite the horrific undertow, here was a man fighting the tides for whatever small degree of personal integrity he could muster.

When I first met him, Harvey was in imminent danger of losing a highly stressful job. His behavior at work had become inappropriately obsessive and ritualistic. Although a leave of absence was suggested, murmuring preoccupations superseded his consideration of a corporate compensation or disability plan. Rather than look into how he could survive, Harvey toyed with the idea of challenging his boss to a wrestling match. He said some vague things about "smearing his weapon." There was no noticeable excitement as he meandered through memories of boyhood and teenage fist fights. In fits, he would clutch at his crotch murmuring about lost power. Clutching represented the enormity of how he had come to experience his life/death struggles. In a near jumble of metaphors, he turned to me directly and emphatically stated that he must protect his strength from the power of the "weak."

Harvey's day dream fragments were filled with images of "falling through insisting cracks." There were no discernible ends to these drops. In the past, it was nightmares which had awakened him. Lately, free falls and collisions melded into his waking hours. To reach bottom, he told me, would be death. Soon after being forced to take a leave of absence from work, he began to fear sleep. He would sit erect for days and nights tapping his hands as if to the beat of marching music.

When most lucid, Harvey referred to himself as "the slimy shark," who, if it were not for the rapids, might have the power to devour other people.

"Why?" I asked.

"To force them to their feet."

"But with such power of your side, how could they then have any feet to stand on?"

We were in a sort of exchange in which we'd each appeared to emphasize a particular view of submergence. The contrast figured into a multifaceted picture of Harvey's confusion.

Images of vying tides and rapids embodied his anxiety. I thought that he might be propelling himself to fight for his own cause. But when this same anxiousness was without imagery, fear and passivity took over. He had become his own "the broken image. . . . An image so contorted and malformed that even tossed from a bridge would produce no further fragments."

In time I became what little projected extension he could cope with. He saw me as some way to composure.

The day he left his job, Harvey became homebound. Just as soon as a bed became available, he entered a psychiatric hospital as a voluntary patient. During his stay in the hospital, our contacts continued over the telephone. He seemed content that his fate was finally in others' hands. Even so, he became restless. An attending psychiatrist had prescribed Haldol, an anti-psychotic medication which he continued to take in varied dosages even after his discharge from the hospital.

His wife Meg was in therapy, but reportedly, her sessions with the woman she referred to as her "counselor" were sporadic and intermittent. With Harvey's permission, I saw her on several occasions as an aid to his resumption of independent living. Meg was more concerned about her own survival. Harvey's three month hospital stay only added to their fundamental marital problems. "Yes," she said, "things had calmed down. But it feels to me like he's either had a lobotomy or that he's even more frightened out of his wits. . . . If he can diminish so completely, what am I to do?" She reported that he most often collapsed in a chair and mumbled to himself. Some of the time it seemed as if he was in shock or seizure. "I find it difficult to distract him," she said, "and I'm frightened that he might strike out at me. . . . When he stands he paces in circles. The repetitiveness nearly drives me crazy. After a while, I try to convince him to sit." I asked her what she thought he might be trying to express by walking in circles. She indicated that he might be tying imaginative knots with his body.

"Do you feel caught in the knots, (i.e., nots)?"

"Maybe," she admitted, "but frankly, he seems scattered and indifferent. The kind of indifference where he's always underfoot, always demanding." She paused. Later she said that she was willing to grant that he'd been under great strain. But there was something about him that had always blinded him to anyone else's needs.

"From what you say," I suggested, "could it be possible that Harvey circles around in some attempt to gather in his world, even if he makes it impossible for anyone to actually relate to him in the process? . . . Perhaps it's not at all unlike his images of the tides, undertows, whirlpools and circling sharks. Autistic children frequently spin around with their hands clutching their genitals or genitalia as if in some sort of an attempt to protect their existences. Harvey had once mentioned that he moved in circles so that he could remain in one piece. Harvey was present during this conversation. It was his way of keeping anyone else in one place."

I once asked him: "Does what you're pacing mean that you have the capacity for seeing people in circles?"

"My wife."

"And why your wife?"

"Without her I'm all out of control."

"A shark out of control could devour people. Then again there are the bigger sharks who are piloted by the smaller ones."

"Since all of this is happening to me happening with me, I suppose I'm both big and small."

"How's that feel?" I asked.

"I'll have to play by more of the rules," he said.

"But you were more involved in the rules than you were in the work. Isn't that why you were forced to go on temporary disability?" I paused. He said nothing. "Was it more important that you knew where everyone was, even more than know where you were at? It takes enormous creativity to look at so many things at once. But hell, you've had to pay for it."

Eventually, Harvey returned to his company. In the meantime, he'd been reassigned. The cast of characters had all but changed. Very little was as he remembered it. His memory had become somewhat blurred. His obsessiveness, now in partial remission, remained a steadying force. Spinning in circles had its proven rewards: "I like being able to keep my eyes on everyone at once."

The return to work remained a tenuous victory.

Therapy proceeded. Harvey gradually recognized his own purposes in translating how he saw things into relatable, if not primitive, frames of reference. In time, he took personal responsibility for his construction of social reality. He termed it his "sensitivity."

The current concern was how to share what needed to be shared in order to survive in what Harvey deemed to be a questionable environment. I took his concern as a direct question. "You've been able to hold on and let go in a way all on your own. You've regularly staved off storms. And while those storms have sometimes had you under, you begin to understand that underlying it all is your personal way of refining your own power and competence. You are unique, which often makes you feel alone and not comparable to anyone else you know."

A World Apart

Maurice Friedman's (1992) cogent description of the isolation/participant quality of the schizophrenic bears citing. "The schizophrenic," according to Friedman,

> . . . even in his desire to have a world of his own apart from the common world, helps to build the common world of speech-with-meaning. His voice cannot be excluded without impoverishing us all. (p. 227)

Psychotic imagery can indeed be regarded as both challenging and crafty. Schizophrenics frequently develop a workable knowledge of their "strangeness." Ultimately, Harvey appreciated the value of his own strange meaning. His imagery, no matter how perilous, served that meaning. From a humanistic perspective, personal authorship and legitimacy are qualities which are to be encouraged. For Harvey, as for others, the task was to reverence himself in his assertiveness and non-assertiveness. If he created the impression that he had little or no identity, then it, too, was necessary to protect what was, for Harvey, most unique about himself.

For Harvey, there was a continuing lessening of the haphazard demonstration of shifting affects. A possible effect of the small amount of the anti-psychotic medication Haldol had been different for Harvey. For many, drugs like Haldol become unfortunate snares, creating an embittered dependency. For him, the effect of Haldol, though he was using it in much reduced doses, had the continuing paradoxical effect of enriching his range of responses to the challenge of sometimes incapacitating circumstances.

None of what ultimately happened to Harvey could simply be regarded as a "cure," even though many terrors had since been abated and the storms of yesterday seemed more in control. Harvey appeared to be less schizophrenic in his basic orientation to reality. All could change at any moment. Schizoid cognition continued to be his mainstay. But for now, he and I were better able to engage in a more dimensional dialogue. Our exchanges took on new challenges; what Laing (1965) properly alluded to as what simply had never happened before in the former transference. At times, Harvey forced himself to be more keenly aware of my constantly reorganized presence. At times, I spoke for him, always careful not to "defeat" his imagery in the process. At other times, he addressed me as someone he was beginning to know better than he had ever known any human being before. I sensed a starting point. A unique relationship had been built.

Despite the deepening of our relationship, suicidal ideation continued. I responded to his suicide threats by emphasizing a universal tendency to prepare for death in any way we can. Self-disclosures were appropriate to our dialogue. I told Harvey that I daily perused the obituary section of the newspaper. "Do you ever see your own name among the dead?" he asked.

"Sometimes," I answered.

"There are times," he said, "that I feel less of a danger dead than alive."

I nodded: "Like no more surprises for you?"

"Yeah, just get it over with."

"Your life, you mean?"

"Not entirely," he replied, "In fact, I don't think I really relish dying. Maybe I will someday, but not for now."

"Could it be," I suggested, "that the equivalent of dying is more like being a nobody without any responsibility? . . . Like a baby?"

"Not at all. Babies have much too much to look forward to."

"And," I was quick to reply, "they probably deal with an awful lot of anxiety, even when they're taken care of just right. You know, like a fear of falling."

"I hate the vision of falling. For me," he said, "it's more like falling to pieces."

"Can you tell me how that happens?"

"Like living in my TV. Sometimes it feels so real, even though I know it isn't. The characters talk specially to me, and then they don't. But I still believe that they do. And they give me survival pointers. They don't always; so I guess, on the whole, I'm pretty frightened of turning the tube on. But I do despite myself."

"Is it that they take away your will?" I asked.

"Well, as I said, they talk right to me. And sometimes I feel I must obey. But obey has come to mean many things to me. I've learned that I can obey one side or the other of their messages."

"So what I hear you say is that if you're not real careful they can make you fall. Seems to me that it's up to you to weigh their impact."

"That's what I mean. And it's not limited to the television. Telephones pressure me. That's one of the reasons I felt tempted to not return to my office. Someone could call, and I can hear the messages in ways they're not intended to be heard."

He suddenly appeared to be dispirited. I waited. "Could it be that they, the people who call and leave messages, any idea that are you really saying something important to yourself at that time? Seems like they are the soundings you most fear. Tell you what, if I were you, I would file any messages for future use. Or else they could be old dispatches, like from your parents, teachers or kids from way back when. Maybe talking about a problem kid? Who knows?" I continued to wait.

Necessary Paranoia

Paranoia is a necessary ingredient in life, and especially important for the schizophrenic. For my part, I find it clinically essential to grant credibility to every paranoid experience. "So just maybe," I continued, "the phone and the TV are also trying to tell you something about the power you are loath to want to take responsibility for?"

(Sometime later) "You said earlier that you do not easily identify yourself with infancy. But I see you're wanting all the background babble and the TV talk to reduce you to a place where you are cared for by being both more or less than anyone else."

Harvey learned from all of the elements of his breakdown. From his experience with the anti-psychotic drug Haldol, he learned not necessarily not to be schizophrenic, but that within his repertoire, he was capable of circumventing crippling anxiety. Likewise, his psychotherapy helped him to appreciate the creative possibilities within the experience of anxiety. He came to know that obsessions, which had frequently removed him from the core of responsibilities, could just as well become the means of mastering them. He could, with some effort, make use of his paranoia in orienting himself to his new assignment. The temptation was to yield to the grandiosity of nothingness in performing the tasks of his new high demanding position (Stern, E. M., 1984).

Non-Existence

Underlying my work with Harvey was my continuing awareness of his drive *not* to be. As a schizophrenic, his identity was hovering between being and not having "been there" and "not yet there." The obsessive walking in circles and the unwillingness not to recline in bed had become his means of engaging his dizziness by not falling into a greater pit of unawareness. Although he was not prepared to die, he was more than willing to allow for social and emotional estrangement, to dislocate from himself. He was, in his mind, an absent presence. I had little desire to fix his predicament. That would have certainly misplaced both of our energies.

In no way did I or do I romanticize the pain of Harvey's memories. Harvey's existence hovered at the melding zones of unrestrained fury, despair and confusing boundaries. Because of this medley, his imagery bordered close to the grotesque. Psychotherapy heals through a recasting of images and memories no matter how despairing they may appear to the unattuned ear. Harvey's images were filled with depression, anxiety, restlessness and paranoid delusions, yet they were at one with his search for significance and meaning. The recital of anger, anguish and terror, many dating back to his earliest years, stimulated our dialog. Though rarely "in touch" with anything beyond his estrangement, he began to hear himself through my recapitulations, I became appreciative of his fear that he had failed simply because he was different. His only hope, probably not at all different from the aspirations of other schizoid and schizophrenic patients, was to win me over to his way even as his attention was otherwise directed. This small task provided Harvey with a necessary modicum of validity.

DANGERS FOR THE THERAPIST

Leslie Farber (1976) notes that prolonged exposure to the schizophrenic can be precarious. And while he in no way suggests that schizophrenia is contagious, he does conclude that the therapist "tends to become something other than the person somewhat he is, or was, or was meant to be" (p. 105). Farber sees the potential for deteriorating relations in the personal life of the therapist. And there is some doubt that therapists who have worked closely with schizophrenics ever truly re/cover the ground they once tread. Undoubtedly this argument, and not the controversy about whether psychotherapy or pharmacology is in the best interest of the psychotic patient, treads the cautions of close therapeutic ties with the schizophrenic.

ADVANTAGES IN TREATING SCHIZOPHRENICS

Therapists who, with experience, respectfully treat psychotic patients, appear more likely to develop the capacity for creating unique intuitive postures. Some are simply more inclined to the language of deep emotional estrangement. It is those few who successfully provide the necessary give-and-take so fundamental in working with the psychotic. But estrangement need not be a final condition. There is, as Eigen (1986) has suggested, a psychotic core underlying the vast range of emotional states and mental disorders. This core may, in my opinion, be a vital signifier for all, those who are schizophrenic and those who are the fellow travelers of schizophrenics. There is, in this core, an insistent need to recognize an inherent tendency to reorder the priorities of being. And since the schizophrenic may be in touch with non-ordinary dimensions of existence, the talking cure for psychosis is a back-and-forth one in which therapist and patient are reshaped, if not transformed, by and through their dialogue.

REFERENCES

Aurelius, M. (1964) *Meditations.* (translated by M. Stainforth) Harmondsworth, Middlesex, England: Penguin Books.

Deinelt, M. (1979) quoted in S. Kopp, *The hanged man.* Palo Alto, CA: Science and Behavior Books (p. 231).

Eigen, M. (1986) *The psychotic core.* Northvale, NJ: Jason Aronson.

Farber, L. (1976) *Lying, despair, jealousy, envy, sex, suicide, drugs, and the good life.* NY: Basic Books.

Friedman, M. (1992) *Religion and psychology: A dialogical approach.* NY: Paragon House Publishers.

Gauquelin, M. (1967) *The cosmic clocks.* NY: Avon Books.

James, W. (1958) *The varieties of religious experience.* New York: The New American Library.

Knight, R. (1993) Converging models of cognitive deficit in schizophrenia. In Dienster, R. (Series Ed.) *Nebraska symposium on motivation,* Vol 31, Lincoln, NE: University of Nebraska Press (pp. 93-156).

Laing, R. D. (1965) Mystification, confusion and conflict. In I. Boszormenyi-Nagi & J. Framo (Eds.) *Intensive family therapy.* NY: Harper & Row.

Magaro, P. (1983) Psychosis and schizophrenia. In Dienster, R. (Series Ed.) *Nebraska symposium on motivation,* Vol. 31, Lincoln, NE: University of Nebraska Press (pp. 157, pp. 230).

May, R. (1983) *The discovery of being: Writings in existential psychology.* New York: Norton.

Pascal, B. (1961) Cited in Ungersma, A. *The search for meaning: A new approach in psychotherapy.* Philadelphia: Westminister Press.

Rank, O. (1929) *The trauma of birth.* NY: Harcourt, Brace & Co.

Schilder, P. (1952) *Psychotherapy.* London: Routledge & Kegan.

Searles H. (1961) Schizophrenia and the inevitability of death. *Psychiatric Quarterly,* 35, pp. 631-655.

Stern, E. M. (1984) Schizophrenic hilarity. *Voices: The Art and Science of Psychotherapy,* 20, 2, pp. 2-8.

Stern, E. M. (1986) Foundations for a soul psychology. In Gibson, K., Lathrop, D. & Stern, E. M. (Eds.) *Carl Jung and Soul Psychology.* NY: Harrington Park Press (pp. 2-7).

Tillich, P. (1957) *Systematic theology,* Vol. 2. Chicago: The University of Chicago Press.

Torrey, E. F. (1995) *Surviving schizophrenia: A manual for consumers and providers* (3rd edition). NY: Harper Perennial.

Walsh, R., Elgin, D., Vaughn, F. and Wilber, K. (1980) Paradigms in collision. In Walsh, R. & Vaughn, F. (Eds.) *Beyond ego.* Los Angeles: J. P. Tarcher (pp. 36-58).

Psychotherapy and the Fear
of Understanding Schizophrenia

Bertram P. Karon
Leighton C. Whitaker

SUMMARY. Understanding schizophrenic persons means facing facts about ourselves, our families, and our society that we do not want to know, or to know again (in the case of repressed feelings and experiences). The central role of terror in producing symptoms, and the genesis and psychological handling of symptoms, including delusions and hallucinations, are briefly described. *[Article copies available from The Haworth Document Delivery Service: 1-800-342-9678.]*

Moral treatment, an early psychologically based treatment for schizophrenics, was tried out, found to be successful, then abandoned (Bockoven, 1972) in favor of harmful somatic treatments (Alexander & Selesnick, 1966; Whitaker, in press). What then was "moral treatment" and why was it replaced by inferior and injurious treatments?

Moral treatment principles were very simple. First of all, no cruelty was permitted. Physical force was permitted only to keep a patient from hurting himself or someone else but not for punishment, not for "negative reinforcement," not for anything else. Harassment, ridicule, and humilia-

---

Bertram P. Karon, PhD, is Professor of Clinical Psychology, Michigan State University, Psychology Research Building, East Lansing, MI 48824-1117.

Leighton C. Whitaker, PhD, is Adjunct Clinical Professor, Institute for Graduate Clinical Psychology. Private Practice address: 220 Turner Road, Wallingford, PA 19086-6037.

[Haworth co-indexing entry note]: "Psychotherapy and the Fear of Understanding Schizophrenia." Karon, Bertram P., and Leighton C. Whitaker. Co-published simultaneously in *The Psychotherapy Patient* (The Haworth Press, Inc.) Vol. 9, No. 3/4, 1996, pp. 23-41; and: *Psychosocial Approaches to Deeply Disturbed Persons* (eds: Peter R. Breggin, and E. Mark Stern) The Haworth Press, Inc., 1996, pp. 23-41. Single or multiple copies of this article are available from The Haworth Document Delivery Service [1-800-342-9678, 9:00 a.m. - 5:00 p.m. (EST)].

23

tion were banned. Hippocrates' principle that if you do not know how to help the patient at least do nothing that will be harmful to the patient, was taken seriously. Second, it was deemed important to keep an accurate case history, which might reveal relevant information about this particular patient and about people with similar disorders. Third, one was to do one's best to understand the patient as an individual human being. Work and social relationships were encouraged as part of normal life.

In our time, psychoanalytic psychotherapy and other psychological treatment modalities for schizophrenia are not fashionable; not because they are not helpful, but because they make the professionals who become therapists, as well as the public at large, so uncomfortable. It is usual to attribute this discomfort to the assumption that schizophrenic people are extremely different from the rest of us. The truth is just the opposite. What makes both professionals and the general public uncomfortable with schizophrenic people is not so much their difference from us, but their similarity. We do not want to know what they have to teach us about the human condition, including our own (Deikman, 1971).

In the 1930s, psychiatrists Harry Stack Sullivan and Frieda Fromm-Reichmann consistently helped schizophrenics. The treatment was arduous, but patients improved. They described their psychoanalytic treatment in their papers and books (Sullivan, 1953; Fromm-Reichmann, 1950). The well-known novel, *I Never Promised You a Rose Garden* (Greenberg, 1964) described that early treatment. The author, who had been a patient of Fromm-Reichmann, used an assumed name, possibly because she was embarrassed. It was only after later novels under her own name became popular that she finally attached her name to this book, which not only describes such treatment but demonstrates the kind of recovery that allows the patient to write so well. Yet, many professionals act as if they have never heard of psychotherapy with schizophrenics or that it has been demonstrated long ago to be unhelpful and inferior to somatic treatment.

Of course, there are economic, sociological, political, ideological, and apparently scientific motives for turning away from understanding schizophrenics. But we would be remiss in ignoring the fundamental emotional bases underlying these motives. The economic, sociological, political, ideological, and "scientific" motives act in concert to maintain a stubborn fear-laden obfuscation of the emotional truths, while serving to rationalize ineffective or even harmful "practical" (in the short run) forms of neglect and mistreatment.

Throughout our professional careers (over 36 and 28 years respectively) we have treated, among other people, schizophrenic patients by psychotherapy. Whenever, in the course of this treatment, something about a schizophrenic person has come to light, it has always illuminated the human condition in general; and whatever psychology has learned about the general human condition has illuminated schizophrenia as well and is helpful in its treatment.

As is well-known, Freud's most important discovery was the unconscious part of the mind which includes the repressed feelings, thoughts, wishes, and memories which are too frightening, guilt-producing, or painful to think about; keeping them repressed saves us pain in the short run. To understand schizophrenic persons is to grasp painful facts about the human condition that we would rather not know, or, more frightening, to be reminded of painful facts we once knew, but repressed.

Even the sociological data about schizophrenia remind us of unpleasant realities. Thus, the disproportionately greater incidence and prevalence of schizophrenic disorders associated with low socioeconomic status, which cannot be accounted for by downward drift, suggests, and psychotherapeutic experience makes vivid, the physical and psychological pain, humiliation, and physical danger associated with being very poor in our society—realities which those of us who are not very poor do not like to perceive or remember. Similarly, schizophrenic disorders are more common among those who are the victims of prejudice and discrimination (e.g., Karon, 1975). Thus, the psychotherapist, to be effective, will often be confronted with the ugliness of economic, racial, ethnic, and religious discrimination which have contributed to these disorders. And the fact that the long-term prognosis for schizophrenics is better in nonliterate cultures (Sartorius, Jablensky, & Shapiro, 1978) reminds us of the relative lack of kindness in our "civilization."

Many schizophrenics have talked about incest, sexual abuse, and physical abuse, but such talk nearly always has been dismissed as the ravings of lunatics. Freud reported that the incest memories specifically of conversion hysterics, related in psychoanalysis, were revealed more often to be fantasies rather than real events, although in many cases, according to Freud, they were undoubtedly real (e.g., Freud, 1917/1977, p. 370). Psychology, psychiatry, and psychoanalysis (but not Freud) falsely generalized that all such memories of patients were only fantasies, since it was believed incest was a rare event. Those therapists and researchers who worked with schizophrenics (e.g., Lidz, 1973) however, reported that the incest "fantasies" related by those patients more often reflected real events, as did their memories of child abuse. The ugly realities of child abuse—psychological, physical, and sexual (including incest)—in our society are only now evident to most mental health professionals. It is now known, for example, that one out of six, and perhaps one out of three, women have been sexually abused (Gagnon, 1965; Finkelhor, 1979; Russell, 1983).

Psychotherapeutic work with schizophrenics revealed that, lacking adequate nurturance, they often wish to be their own mother. This wish, consciously or unconsciously, may underlie many symptoms (e.g., rocking, sucking, male patients wishing to be a woman, irrational needs to feed [literally or symbolically] oneself or others). Later, Kestenberg (1975), on the basis of her observation and treatment of children, reported that at the age of two nearly every child goes through a stage where he or she wants to be a mother. Girls want to be a mother to a little girl, and boys want to be a mother to a little boy, so it is clear whose mother they want to be. Schizophrenics simply continue this need into adulthood.

In order to help a postpartum schizophrenic (Rosberg & Karon, 1959) it was necessary to learn (in her psychotherapy) about the fantasy that anything that filled the body was food. But Michel-Hutmacher (1955) reported that normal children under seven regularly reported that belief. Again, one can understand how schizophrenics, lacking nurturant satisfaction, would retain that belief as a kind of wish-fulfillment as well as a cognitive or perceptual failure in differentiation. One implication, as Sechehaye (1951) has so well demonstrated, is that fulfillment of the need by a therapist skilled enough to devise a strategy that takes into account both the patient's need and fear can result in cognitive and perceptual clarity.

One schizophrenic patient (Rosberg & Karon, 1958) revealed clearly, and other schizophrenic patients confirmed, the existence of a terrifying fantasy of having the inside of your body emptied out and drained, a terror originating in early infancy, and augmented or diminished by later experiences. This fantasy takes various symptomatic forms, including in some male patients that of a fear of being emptied or drained through the penis, which is often experienced as more frightening than castration. Thus some patients attempt to cut off their penises as the lesser evil. The therapist's knowledge of that fantasy allows one to recognize the subtle evidence of it that occurs in some relatively normal men whose impotence is derived from this fear and, consequently, to help these nonschizophrenic impotent patients as well.

THE PATIENT'S TERROR AND THERAPIST REACTION

What happens when a therapist talks to a schizophrenic? Usually the therapist at least feels uncomfortable, depressed, and/or angry, because the patient doesn't react the way the therapist wants him or her to react; the patient often does not show the therapist respect. What the therapist knows does not seem to work. But, in addition, the therapist feels scared and isn't sure why. Despite their personal therapy and professional training, mental health professionals do not like to experience those feelings or affects any more than anyone else does. It is not an accident that the most illuminating discussions of negative countertransference have come from therapists who have worked with schizophrenics (e.g., Searles, 1965). Sometimes the therapist may, all too successfully, empathize with the schizophrenic patient's terror and tend to withdraw in terror just like the patient.

One of the reasons for these uncomfortable feelings on the part of the therapist talking to schizophrenic people is that these are their feelings communicated, as it were, to the therapist. One of the great mistakes made in evaluating schizophrenia (probably because of our fear of empathy and contagion, a mistake that even Eugen Bleuler made) is to assume that because they look as if they have no feeling or affect that they have no feelings. A common mistake in assessment is for the examiner to report lack of affect instead of lack of affect expression. In fact, schizophrenic persons have very intense feelings, i.e., affects, although they may mask or even deny them. The primary or most basic affect is fear or, more precisely, terror: that is, a seemingly all-pervasive, all-defeating fear that is by its nature so difficult to describe as to be ineffable and thus an ultimately lonely and alienating experience.

A man who appeared to be in a coma when picked out of a gutter by the police was brought to a hospital where he continued not to move or speak for three days. Meanwhile, exhaustive physical tests showed no physical pathology. After an hour with a psychologist who treated him as a terrified person, he became quite communicative. The turning point in coming out of his "coma" was when the psychologist asked what he was afraid of, to which he replied, "Everything, everything is dangerous." The psychologist guaranteed him of several safe people and situations much as a parent might do. He then talked easily and ate a meal.

Human beings are not easily able to tolerate chronic, massive terror. All of the symptoms of schizophrenia may be understood as manifestations of chronic terror or defenses against the terror. The chronic terror tends to hide other feelings. Nonetheless, the schizophrenic frequently experiences, in addition to fear—whether chronically or intermittently—anger, hopelessness, loneliness, and humiliation.

Fundamentally, we do not want to know about schizophrenia because we do not want to feel terror at that intensity. All of us have the potential for schizophrenic symptoms if there is enough stress; the only differences seem to lie in the quantity and qualitative nature of the necessary stress.

In World War II the word "schizophreniform" psychosis was used to describe patients who looked just like schizophrenics in every way, but "couldn't" be schizophrenics because the patients got better. One battlefield situation that apparently provoked these "schizophreniform" reactions in every soldier was very simple: an infantryman was under fire. He dug a hole and, since the enemy was trying to kill him, as soon as the hole was barely big enough, he got into it. The enemy kept shooting at him; he had no place to go without being killed. He urinated on himself, and he defecated on himself. When his rations were gone, he did not eat and did not drink. If this stress lasted for three or more consecutive days, until the shooting stopped, every soldier who survived looked like a classic schizophrenic (Grinker & Spiegel, 1965). But, if the soldier had been a reasonably healthy person before this trauma, security and rest almost always led to a spontaneous recovery. In those days they "knew" schizophrenics never got better so, therefore, it could not really be schizophrenia; hence, the diagnosis "schizophreniform" reaction. Yet the key to understanding schizophrenic reactions lay in those observations.

THE THERAPEUTIC ALLIANCE

Because of the intensity of the terror and the bleakness of the patient's expectations, therapists do not want to know what the patient experiences. But without such understanding, without being able to tolerate such feelings, and without being able to be hopeful about the outcome, no therapeutic alliance is possible. Yet psychotherapy research in general reveals that with any type of psychotherapy and any patient, the single best predictor of outcome is whether there is a therapeutic alliance. That is, does the patient feel that the therapist and the patient are on the same side, and that the therapist wants to be and is capable of being helpful? Many neurotics bring enough positive elements from their experience of their parents to their initial therapeutic transference to make it strongly positive and the therapeutic alliance is easily achieved. Schizophrenics, on the other hand, usually have had so many bad experiences with other people that forming a therapeutic alliance is rarely automatic. Sometimes it is achievable early in therapy, and in other cases achieving a therapeutic alliance may be the major focus of work for a long time. It is important to recognize, however, that it is up to the therapist and not the patient to make the therapeutic alliance possible.

Insofar as other important people in the patient's life, including parents and treatment professionals, may have been hurtful, uncaring, inadequate, or pessimistic, ambiguity on the part of the therapist will lead to the patient filling in the ambiguity by seeing the therapist as hurtful, uncaring, inadequate, or pessimistic. The therapist should not be ambiguous, but clear that he or she wants to help the patient, wants to understand, that the patient is helpable, and that it will only take hard work. Since patients are afraid that other people want to hurt them, they frequently will not communicate clearly even what they understand. Patients will therefore not be surprised that you do not understand everything; they will be impressed that you understand anything, particularly if it is something no one else has understood.

It is not the therapist's accurate understanding or empathy for the patients which is curative, nor is that what the patients perceive when they say we understand them; rather it is our attempt to accurately understand them which is curative and which they perceive as understanding. It is a benign trauma. No one has ever really tried hard to understand them, and how unpleasant their subjective lives have been.

The patients frequently do not communicate even that you are helping them, for fear that it will be used against them. Therefore, the therapist sometimes must work with an act of faith that if you do reasonable things long enough the patient will get better, and notice small changes, or get feedback from the family or ward staff, or notice that when the patient complains of new problems, they are often such that the patient can only have these problems if other more serious problems had been overcome.

Sometimes all one has to do is ask, "What seems to be the trouble? How can I help you?" If you take seriously what they ask, and help them, even if it is not with what you think is the major problem, the basis for an alliance develops.

For many patients it is useful to directly address the terror by saying, "I won't let anyone kill you." While patients may be skeptical of your ability to do so, they are impressed that you know with what they are concerned, and hope that you mean it. Since for most patients the life-threatening danger is now intra-psychic, only a therapist can save them. For some, however, there are real dangers in the outside world and it is critical that one help them think about dangers realistically, and cope with the dangers whether those are reality dangers over which the patient has no control but with which he or she must cope, or reality dangers which the patient has helped to create, or delusional dangers.

Some patients seem so formidable that even the decision "I won't run screaming from the room" means that the therapy has already begun.

CLINICAL EXPERIENCE OF PSYCHOLOGICAL CAUSALITY

Clinical experience leads one to be skeptical of genetic factors for schizophrenia. Of course, hospital records and superficial examinations often make the disorder seem uncaused. But if one dares to listen carefully, the disorder always makes psychological sense and seems inevitable in terms of the life as experienced.

A favorite example was provided by psychiatry residents at a state hospital who endured a seminar with Karon on psychotherapy with schizophrenics, which made them uncomfortable since they were told that shock treatment and psychosurgery were destructive, and medication was of limited benefit. They were encouraged to talk to their patients. That was not what the rest of their supervisors told them. The residents, in reaction, asked the instructor to interview a patient.

Most schizophrenics are not dangerous, but the residents chose someone with a history of repeatedly assaulting strange men, who himself was big, muscular, and moved very fast. The patient had been hospitalized for ten years, but there was nothing in the case records which would account for his disorder. The only apparent major stresses were that he was poor, his father was an alcoholic, he developed a speech disorder (stutter) which did not respond to speech therapy as an adolescent. He also reported a venereal disease in the army (whose site was in his mouth), just before his first assault on a stranger.

He was grossly incoherent and, when he became coherent, he stuttered very badly. All the residents could have done to choose a more difficult psychotherapy prospect would be to choose someone who didn't speak English at all! The lecturer insisted that the residents sit in the same room during the interview, knowing they had never been that close to anybody who moved that fast or was that dangerous.

In our value system, which most patients share, one deals first with homicidal danger; secondly, suicidal danger; and thirdly, anything else. This patient would creep up behind other patients and choke them. The attendants would see feet waving in the air. The patient had not killed anyone (he dropped the victim when the victim was unconscious), but the attendants were worried that he might kill someone.

Therefore, the interviewer kept bringing up this symptom during the first session. Finally, the patient and he worked out what seemed to be going on. When he was a little boy, his mother, for minor offenses like not eating, would put a cloth around his neck and choke him. This seemed to be the correct psychological reconstruction, since after that first session he stopped choking other patients. (It is a useful clinical rule of thumb that when you get a dramatic improvement in a symptom, you are probably doing the right thing.) Now this is not the kind of difficulty with which even people with difficult mothers have had to cope.

A second fact came to light in a transference reaction. The patient began a therapy hour by yelling, "Why did you do it to me, Dad?" It is not difficult to recognize a transference reaction when a schizophrenic patient calls the therapist "daddy" or "mommy."

"What did I do?"

"You know what you did!"

When asked how old he was, he said, "You know I was eight years old." Bit by bit he revealed that "you" had come home drunk and anally raped him. This was not an ordinary alcoholic father.

The patient's terrible stutter was also revealed to have an extraordinary cause. In the middle of his stutter there were words in Latin. When asked if he had been an altar boy, he said, "You swallow a snake, and then you stutter. You mustn't let anyone know." He was extremely ashamed and guilty. Apparently, he had performed fellatio on a priest.

He was reassured that it was all right, and it was interpreted orally, "Anyone as hungry as you were would have done the same thing." (It is a common finding with schizophrenic patients that much of what seems sexual really has to do with orality, that is, infantile feelings, survival, and the early mother-child relationship. A penis, for example, may represent a mother's breast, and the breast represent love.)

At that point the stuttering stopped. When he started to stutter in later sessions, it was only necessary to repeat the interpretation and the stuttering immediately ceased.

But look at this poor man's life. He turned to mother, and mother was terrible. If mother is terrible, one ordinarily turns to father, but his father was terrible. He turned to God, and the priest was destructive. Would that not drive anyone insane? Yet examination of ten years of ordinary hospital records revealed no basis for his psychosis.

Of course, most parents of schizophrenics are not consciously destructive people, but often admirable people who will go to great lengths to attempt to get help for their children. Sometimes the destructive life experiences have nothing to do with the parents at all; in other instances hurtful parenting is the result of bad professional advice, the repetition of bad parenting that they endured from their own idealized parents, or the result of unconscious defenses of which they are unaware and consequently uncontrollable until brought into awareness.

UNDERSTANDING THE CATATONIC STUPOR

Let us consider what can be learned about the human condition from the most bizarre symptoms of schizophrenia. Take the catatonic stupor, the man or woman who sits in the corner and does not move. They are either absolutely rigid or they may be waxily flexible. They may stay in one position for hours or for days.

Fromm-Reichmann (1950) reported a long time ago that catatonic patients see and hear everything that is going on around them even though they do not react. They look like they are in a stupor, but they are not. They feel as if they will die if they move. Fromm-Reichmann understood this because the patients told her when they finally came out of the stupor.

Some years ago, Ratner (Ratner, Karon, VandenBos, & Denny, 1981) investigated animals in a state that used to be called animal hypnosis.

If one turns an animal upside down and presses it, it becomes rigid or waxily flexible. Rabbits, lions, tigers, alligators, 70 species of birds, fish, octopuses, in fact, just about every species of animal, fish, bird and insect tested show this response. The major exceptions are pet dogs and cats, and laboratory rats in a laboratory where they had been handled gently every day. While sometimes referred to as animal hypnosis, it is not hypnosis–there is no verbal induction, and the animals do not obey commands. But the animal will not move even if great pain is inflicted. After the passage of time the animals come into rapid violent motion unpredictably, which is like human catatonic excitement.

Classical conditioning experiments, pairing two stimuli while the animal is rigid, leads to learning that can be demonstrated after they come out of the state, so they are fully conscious of external stimuli. In fact, it is identical with the catatonic stupor.

Ratner discovered its meaning. Most animals are prey for some predator. Every species has a species-specific sequence of behaviors when it is under attack by a predator–sham death, cries of distress to warn the others in the group, etc. The last stage for every species seems to be this state of rigidity. Most predators, if they are not hungry, will kill their prey and save it for later. Some predators will not even attack something that does not move, but most predators will. When the animal goes into this catatonic-like state, most predators act as if they think it is dead. In an experiment with ferrets and frogs, a ferret, for example, ate the eye out of one frog in this state and the frog did not flinch. The ferret crunched up the foreleg of another in its teeth, and it did not flinch either. In this experiment with ferrets and frogs, 70 percent of the frogs survived. According to Ratner, if even 30 percent survive to one mating, the effect on evolution is massive.

So the catatonic stupor is a life and species preservative strategy that is built into just about all living animals, including human beings. The biological evidence is consistent with the clinical evidence from somebody like Fromm-Reichmann who actually listened to her patients. That needs to be said because there are many "experts" on schizophrenia who have never listened to any of their patients for more than half an hour.

But we do not want to know that you and I would go catatonic if we were terrified enough. Nor do we want to know what it feels like to be that terrified.

HALLUCINATIONS

As with the catatonic stupor, every other schizophrenic symptom is a universal human potentiality. Take hallucinations, the most dramatic symptom of all. Schizophrenic patients as well as professionals like to say that nobody understands hallucinations. But hallucinations are entirely understandable by Freud's (1900/1950, 1916/1935, 1933) theories of dreams, with a few additions. Today, the concept of the collective unconscious seems scientifically untenable; it was based on the then-accepted biological theory of the inheritance of acquired characteristics, no longer acceptable to biologists. There is no evidence of universal symbols; there are only symbols which are frequently used with a given meaning, but there are always people who will use any symbol with an entirely different meaning.

Unlike most people, schizophrenics hallucinate while they are wide awake. Everyone hallucinates when asleep. Dreams may take any sensory modality, but the predominant experience is visual. Schizophrenics also may hallucinate in any sensory modality, but the predominant modality is auditory. Whatever other hallucinations they have, they almost always hear voices. That is different from toxic psychoses where the hallucinations are primarily visual. (That is why LSD research was irrelevant. LSD produces phenomena which are primarily visual, like any other toxic psychosis, but not at all like schizophrenia.)

Why predominantly auditory hallucinations? Because basically schizophrenia is an interpersonal disorder. If someone is blind, they are more physically incapacitated than someone who is deaf. In terms of the probability of emotional disorders, someone who is deaf is more likely to have emotional problems caused by it, because it tends to cut them off from people.

But is the capacity to hallucinate while wide awake restricted to schizophrenics? Not at all. It is well known that starving people start seeing food. It is a human capacity if the motivation is strong enough; luckily, most of us will never be desperate enough to have to hallucinate. A trivial example illustrates the meaning of hallucinations. In the middle of a therapy session, a patient asked, "What's that bell?"

"I didn't hear a bell."

"Well, I did."

"It may well be. There are a lot of funny noises in this building. I work here all the time and maybe, like a lighthouse keeper, I just don't pay attention to them anymore. What did the bell sound like?"

"It sounded like a telephone bell, only very loud."

"That's surprising. A telephone bell I would have heard. What comes to mind when you think of a telephone bell?"

"Trying to get through to somebody."

"I think I know what's happening. I've been talking about what I thought was important, but you know I'm off somewhere and you wish I would get through to you and talk about what is really going on here."

And then the patient smiled. She was too intimidated to tell the therapist he did not understand and ask why he was talking about irrelevancies when there were some things that were important. The most she could do was wish that somehow he would get through to her; even that was too frightening to deal with consciously, so she had to have it come through in disguise, as a hallucination.

DELUSIONS

As mentioned above, attempts to understand delusions would have led to considering incest, sexual abuse of children, and physical abuse of children as serious problems in our society. What else do we not want to know?

There are four bases for delusions. The most important source of delusions is Freud's concept of transference: reliving feelings, fantasies, and experiences from the past with no awareness that it is the past. Of course, Freud thought schizophrenics did not form transference. He was mistaken because he did not talk to schizophrenics. According to people who knew him, Freud said schizophrenic patients scared him. He certainly had enough work to do without schizophrenic patients. But even Freud's inferences are unlikely to be accurate unless they are based on clinical observations.

Freud originally thought of transference as a phenomenon occurring only in psychoanalysis, as the chief resistance, which by understanding he was able to transform into its most potent therapeutic tool. Ferenczi (1909/1950) first pointed out, and Freud accepted, that transference, like other resistances, was a defense used to cope in ordinary life. What was unique about transference in therapy was not its occurrence, but that it was studied.

However, the transference reactions of normals and neurotics are sufficiently subtle and realistic that one need not be upset by being reminded how pervasively we re-create and re-experience our past. But schizophrenics, if listened to, are not subtle in their transference.

Nor are the specific contents of their transference matters of which most of us wish to be reminded. It is not pleasant to be reminded of the varieties of misery which are inflicted on children in our society. Even more troubling than the awareness of obviously hurtful or neglectful treatment of children is the insight that parents of admirable character and with the very best of intentions, may harm their children, either because their hurtful interactions are unconscious (Karon, 1960; Meyer & Karon, 1967) or because the parents are misinformed about the consequences of their actions.

The most famous example of a history of such hurtfulness, albeit unintentional, is Schreber, a judge in Germany, a paranoid schizophrenic man who was declared legally sane. After he left the hospital, he wrote a book (Schreber 1903/1955) exposing the plot against him. Freud read the book and had some important insights, but missed the transference.

Schreber claimed that God put metal bands around his head and his chest and tightened them "lovingly" until it hurt. Further, God wanted to castrate him and make him a woman.

Schreber's father (Niederland, 1959, 1960, 1972, 1984) was a world famous pediatrician who wrote books on how to raise children. His advice included advocating that "bad habits," by which he meant masturbation, should be punished immediately and they will disappear by the age of four, never recur and leave no bad after effects. He knew because he had done this with both of his sons. One committed suicide, and the other became the most famous paranoid schizophrenic ever.

The father believed that exercise and posture were very important for children. To improve their posture, he invented chairs, tables, and beds with rods and metal rings that went around the head and around the chest to make the child sit up straight and lie absolutely straight. He said he used them "lovingly." We would probably consider them torture devices today. He even advocated devices to discourage masturbation consisting of metal rings with small spikes on the inside which would pierce the child's penis if he had an erection.

What God did in Schreber's delusions was what Schreber's real father actually did to Schreber as a child. What psychiatrist would even consider the possibility that a world famous pediatrician could have done such terrible things? But remember, his father was not intending to torture Schreber; his father thought all of this was good for the child.

To use a more contemporary example, a young woman alarmed the hospital staff by repeatedly cutting and burning herself. When asked about her religion, she said, "I was raised a Catholic."

"Oh, you were raised a Catholic, but you're not now."

"Actually, I'm a Satanist."

"Why don't you tell me about it."

"I used to feel I had to save people. I had to save all the people in Beirut."

"That's a marvelous image. Beirut, that's a marvelous image. You know who the people in Beirut are, don't you?"

She started to say yes and then she said, "Well, no."

"What's Beirut? Beirut is a city where people are killing each other, and then they declare peace. But when you look, they are still killing each other. Then they find out why they are killing each other, and then deal with those problems and solve them; but they go on killing each other. Then they have a truce, but still go on killing each other. What a marvelous image—your family must have been like that."

She became very interested at that point. "Satan says that if I hurt myself, he'll keep me with him. That's what he says."

She was very scared. She described Satan's voice and his appearance. She described his face in considerable detail. When asked whether she knew anybody who looked like that, she thought and said, "Yes; he doesn't look like it now, but he used to."

"Who?"

"My father."

Indeed, according to later information from the family, it turns out her father used to beat her mother, and her mother eventually left the house. One can understand a little girl's belief that pain is the price of not being abandoned.

That hallucination disappeared. All one had to do was to ask the patient to describe her experience and ask what it could possibly mean.

The second source of delusions was described by Freud (1911/1950) on the basis of insights derived from his reading of Schreber's book. As is widely cited, Freud derived many paranoid delusions from the fear of homosexuality as different ways of contradicting the implicit guilt-producing feeling (for a man), "I love him." Thus, I do not love him, I love me—megalomania; I do not love him, I love her—erotomania; I do not love him (using projection), she loves him—delusional jealousy; I do not love him (using projection), he loves me—the delusional threat of being endangered by homosexuals; I do not love him (using reaction formation), I hate him—irrational hatred; or, most common, I do not love him (using reaction formation), I hate him, but I cannot hate him for no reason, so (using projection) he hates me, that is why I hate him, and if I hate him, obviously I do not love him—delusional feelings of persecution.

However, secondary sources almost never mention one part of Freud's insight that is most meaningful and essential for therapeutic effectiveness. In the language of libido theory, Freud said that the patient with schizophrenia feels withdrawn from emotional relatedness to everybody. Consequently, he wants to be able to relate to someone again. In addition to the hunger for approval from the father is the fact that people of the same sex are more like us than the opposite sex, and, in growing up, it is usual to feel comfortable in relating closely to peers of the same sex before becoming comfortable with the opposite sex. When one feels withdrawn from everybody, there is a strong urge to get close to people of the same sex. Unfortunately, the patient fearfully interprets this self-curative tendency as "homosexuality."

But is this different from the normal adolescent, who is having trouble with the opposite sex? Time spent with friends of the same sex leads to becoming more comfortable with people and with the opposite sex. This is the normal developmental sequence. With normals and neurotics, too, the fear of homosexuality leads to withdrawing from friends of the same sex, and that makes relating to the other sex even more difficult. Hence, the generally useful advice for adolescents (or adults) having trouble with the opposite sex is to spend more time with same sex friends, instead of withdrawing from them. This usually makes relating to the opposite sex easier.

Even the specific dynamics of paranoid feelings as defenses are mirrored in the dynamics of some similar feelings in people who are not schizophrenics.

It is usually helpful to let schizophrenic patients with symptoms based on the fear of homosexuality know that their fear of being homosexual is unfounded (if, as is usually the case, it is unfounded). They are simply lonely, that their loneliness is normal, and that we all need friends of both sexes. Unless they have had a meaningful and benign homosexual relationship, schizophrenics are not helped by reassurances concerning the increased acceptability of homosexuality, but they always feel understood when their therapist talks of loneliness.

Of course, Freud's views on paranoid delusions have been criticized, fairly and unfairly. The fair criticism is that they account for only some delusions, not all. The unfair criticism is that persecutors in the delusions of women are usually men. But the first to point out this apparent contradiction was Freud (1915/1957) noting that, when first psychotic, the persecutor is female and is changed to a male persecutor as a later development.

This illustrates the general human condition that feelings about men are not necessarily based on experiences with men, nor are feelings about women necessarily based on experiences with women.

The third basis for delusions is that some families actually teach strange ideas. The study of schizophrenic patients (Lidz, 1973) reveals how human beings depend on their families to teach them the categories of thought and the meaning of those categories. Children (and adults) assume that other people use concepts in the same way, unless confronted with understandable contradictions. For example, if a person believes "I love you" includes in its meaning "I hurt you, physically assault you, occasionally even try to kill you," that person is unlikely ever to be able to relate closely to another in a loving relationship.

It has been noted that families with disturbed children have a tendency to discourage the use of people outside the family as sources of information and corrective identification. Patients from very disturbed families who do not become schizophrenic are inevitably found to have remedied the defects in their nuclear families with relationships outside that family. This is a normal mechanism. Nobody ever had a perfect mother or father, nor can parents provide every kind of nurturance needed. Most children, as well as adults use people outside the family to correct any problems in their family.

When parents interfere with this mechanism, any problem in the family is enormously magnified in its destructive impact. The parents, of course, do not do this to be hurtful; they are unaware that it has any harmful consequences. Indeed, they may even believe that it is good for the child. Parents who discourage extra-familial identifications are spared the normal discomfort of having their values and beliefs challenged by their children. But these challenges, whether or not communicated overtly, partially shield the child from the impact of the inevitable parental mistakes.

The last basis for delusions is the general human need for a more or less systematic explanation of our world.

Most people share similar systematic understandings. One who believes the world is flat is normal if the year is 1400, and is suspect if the year is 1992. The belief is the same; it is the relationship to others' beliefs that makes it normal or suspect. In our pluralistic modern era, one is not considered mentally ill if there is an obvious basis for a different understanding. Thus, a fundamentalist usually does not consider mentally ill those of us who take evolution seriously; he understands that such people take biology, geology, and physics seriously but do not realize the "truth" that God created fossils as fossils.

Schizophrenic people have had strange experiences. In part, their symptoms are strange experiences by ordinary standards. In addition, their lives often include unusual real events. Therefore, their systematic explanations of their world seem strange. But they demonstrate a need to be as realistic as their anxieties permit. Insofar as discrepancies between their understanding and reality become apparent to them, and as dynamic balances change, the patients continually revise their understanding.

The more intelligent patients are more apt to develop a systematic understanding that is adequate enough to obviate the need for more deteriorated symptoms and, hence, to be diagnosed as paranoid or paranoid schizophrenic. The less intelligent are less likely to develop as functionally adequate a "paranoid system."

Because the paranoid system is not an abnormal process, but a normal process used to cope with unusual problems, it is possible for a nonfrightened, nonhumiliating therapist to share the patient's systematic understanding, to respectfully call attention to inconsistencies, and to helpfully supplement the patient's understanding with the therapist's knowledge of the world, other people and, more importantly, of the workings of the human mind.

A PATIENT'S SUMMARY

The best description of what it feels like to be schizophrenic came from a catatonic man whom it took eight weeks of psychotherapy (without medication) to get out of the hospital and back to work. One of his symptoms was bowing. When asked why he bowed, he said, "I don't bow."

"Yes, you do."

"No, I don't bow."

"Wait a minute. You do this [the therapist bowed]. This is bowing; you bow."

"No, I don't bow."

"But you do this."

"That's not bowing."

"What is it?"

"It's balancing."

"What are you balancing?"

"Emotions."

"What emotions?"

"Fear and loneliness."

That is, when he was lonely, he wanted to get close to people (so he leaned forward). When he got close to people, he got scared and had to pull away (so he straightened up). But then he was lonely again.

Balancing between fear and loneliness is the best description of what it feels like to be schizophrenic. But that is what the rest of us do not want to understand.

REFERENCES

Alexander, F. G. & Selesnick, S. T. (1966). *The history of psychiatry.* New York: Harper & Row.

Bockoven, J. S. (1972). *Moral treatment in community mental health.* New York: Springer.

Deikman, A. J. (1971). Phenothiazines and the therapist's fear of identification. *Humanistic Psychology, 11,* 196-200.

Ferenczi, S. (1950). Introjection and transference. *Sex in psychoanalysis.* New York: Brunner/Mazel, 35-93. (Original work published 1909)

Finkelhor, D. H. (1979). *Sexually victimized children.* New York: Free Press.

Freud, S. (1933). *New introductory lectures on psychoanalysis.* New York: Norton.

Freud, S. (1935). *A general introduction to psychoanalysis.* New York: Liveright. (Original work published 1916)

Freud, S. (1950). *The interpretation of dreams.* New York: Macmillan. (Original work published 1900)

Freud, S. (1950). Psychoanalytic notes upon an autobiographical account of a case of paranoia (dementia paranoids). *Collected papers, 3,* 316-357. London: Hogarth and the Institute for Psychoanalysis. (Original work published in 1911)

Freud, S. (1957). A case of paranoia counter to psychoanalytic theory. *Complete psychological works, 14,* 262-300, London: Hogarth. (Original work published 1915)

Freud, S. (1977). *Introductory lectures on psychoanalysis.* (J. Strachey, Trans.) New York: Norton. (Original work published 1917)

Fromm-Reichmann, F. (1950). *Principles of intensive psychotherapy.* Chicago: University of Chicago Press.

Gagnon, J. H. (1965). Female child victims of sex offense. *Sexual problems, 13,* 176-192.

Greenberg, J. (1964). *I never promised you a rose garden.* New York: Holt, Rinehart, & Winston.

Grinker, K. R. & Spiegel, J. P. (1965). *Men under stress.* New York: McGraw-Hill.

Karon, B. P. (1960). A clinical note on the significance of an "oral" trauma. *Journal of Abnormal and Social Psychology, 61,* 480-481.

Karon, B. P. (1975). *Black scars.* New York: Springer.

Karon, B. P., & VandenBos, G. R. (1981). *Psychotherapy of schizophrenia: The treatment of choice.* New York: Aronson.

Kestenberg, J. (1975). *Children and parents: Psychoanalytic studies in development.* New York: Jason Aronson.

Lidz, T. (1973). *The origin and treatment of schizophrenic disorders.* New York: Basic Books.

Meyer, R. G., & Karon, B. P. (1967). The schizophrenogenic mother concept and the TAT. *Psychiatry, 30,* 173-179.

Michel-Hutmacher, R. (1955). Das korperinnere in der vorstellung der kinder. *Schweirische Zeitschrift fuer Psychologie und ihre Anwendungen, 14,* 1-26.

Niederland, W. G. (1959). Schreber: Father and son. *Psychoanalytic Quarterly, 11,* 151-169.

Niederland, W. G. (1960). Schreber's father. *Journal of the American Psychoanalytic Association, 8,* 492-499.

Niederland, W. G. (1972). The Schreber case sixty years later. *International Journal of Psychiatry, 10,* 79-84.

Niederland, W. G. (1984). The Schreber case: Psychoanalytic profile of a paranoid personality. Hillsdale, N.J.: *Analytic Press,* xvi, 180 p.: ill. 23 cm.

Ratner, S. G., Karon, B. P., VandenBos, G. R., & Denny, M. R. (1981). The adaptive significance of the catatonic stupor in humans and animals from an evolutionary perspective. *Academic Psychology Bulletin, 3,* 273-279.

Rosberg, J., & Karon, B. P. (1958). The oedipus complex in an apparently deteriorated case of schizophrenia. *Journal of Abnormal and Social Psychology, 57,* 221-225.

Rosberg, J., & Karon, B. P. (1959). A direct analytic contribution to the understanding of post-partum psychosis. *Psychiatric Quarterly, 33,* 296-304.

Russell, D. E. H. (1983). The incidence and prevalence of intrafamilial and extrafamilial sexual abuse of female children. *Child abuse and neglect, 7,* 133-146.

Sartorius, N., Jablensky, A., & Shapiro, R. (1978). Cross-cultural differences in the short-term prognosis of schizophrenic psychoses. *Schizophrenia bulletin, 4,* 102-113.

Schreber, D. P. (1955). *Memoirs of my recent illness.* (I. Macalping and R. A. Hunter, Trans.) London: Dawson. (Original work published 1903)

Searles, H. F. (1965). *Collected papers on schizophrenia and related subjects.* New York: International Universities Press.

Sechehaye, M. A. (1951). *Symbolic realization.* New York: International Universities Press.

Sullivan, H. S. (1953). *Schizophrenia as a human process.* New York: Norton.

Whitaker, L. (in press). *Assessment of schizophrenia disorders; sense and nonsense.* New York: Plenum.

Soteria:
A Therapeutic Community
for Psychotic Persons

Loren R. Mosher

SUMMARY. A non-medical, non-hospital, non-professional, home-like, minimal medication program for newly diagnosed psychotic persons is described. It is based on moral treatment principles and the tradition of intensive inter-personal intervention with psychosis. Research established that this program was as, or more effective than hospital based, medication dependent, professionally delivered treatment for this subset of psychotic persons. *[Article copies available from The Haworth Document Delivery Service: 1-800-342-9678.]*

INTRODUCTION AND OVERVIEW

In the spring of 1971, a two-story, 12-room, 1912-vintage, wooden house on a busy thoroughfare in San Jose, California, became a second generation Kingsley Hall of London. True to its heritage, Soteria House sat in the midst of a multiethnic working class neighborhood with a number of advantages over its East London parent. First, substantial numbers of college students and former state hospital patients lived in this designated poverty area. Hence transience and deviance were not unknown.

Loren R. Mosher, MD, is Chief Medical Director (Psychiatry) in the Department of Health and Human Services, Adult Mental Health and Substance Abuse Services, Montgomery County, 401 Hungerford Drive, Suite 500, Rockville, MD 20850. The author is also Clinical Professor of Psychiatry, Uniformed Services University of the Health Sciences, Bethesda, MD 20814.

[Haworth co-indexing entry note]: "Soteria: A Therapeutic Community for Psychotic Persons." Mosher, Loren R. Co-published simultaneously in *The Psychotherapy Patient* (The Haworth Press, Inc.) Vol. 9, No. 3/4, 1996, pp. 43-58; and: *Psychosocial Approaches to Deeply Disturbed Persons* (eds: Peter R. Breggin, and E. Mark Stern) The Haworth Press, Inc., 1996, pp. 43-58. Single or multiple copies of this article are available from The Haworth Document Delivery Service [1-800-342-9678, 9:00 a.m. - 5:00 p.m. (EST)].

Second, painting the exterior of the house and replanting its rundown yard helped win acceptance in the community. Third, my London experience convinced me that the house and its staff should attempt to conform to neighborhood social norms. In contrast, the community surrounding Kingsley Hall was instrumental in closing it.

Into this comfortable six bedroom home came—for three to six months—a group of young, unmarried persons newly diagnosed and labeled as having schizophrenia. Six could be accommodated at any one time. The nonprofessional staff also lived there to provide a simple, home-like, safe, warm, supportive, unhurried, tolerant, and unintrusive social environment. Soteria staff believed sincere human involvement and understanding were critical to healing interactions with clients. The project's purpose was to find out whether this type of milieu was as effective in promoting recovery from madness as that provided in a nearby general hospital's psychiatric ward, which was oriented toward using antipsychotic drugs. Ordinarily, the patients assigned to Soteria House receive no antipsychotic drug for six weeks after entry. The staff believed it might take that long before important relationships could form and before the special qualities of the culture there could be meaningfully transmitted. If no healing were evident in six weeks, patients were given a trial of tranquilizers on a case-by-case basis (about 20% received such trials). In contrast, all of the hospital-treated comparison cases received high doses of neuroleptic drugs.

BACKGROUND

Although the author's experiences at Kingsley Hall were important to the development of the Soteria project, difficulties encountered with the treatment of psychosis in hospital settings also provided a major impetus for a home where schizophrenics live through their psychosis with a non-professional staff. To wit, even well staffed "progressive" hospitals invariably have institutional characters which create barriers to establishing relationships which could maximally facilitate recovery from psychosis. The "barrier" characteristics (present to varying degrees in different settings) are:

Theoretical Model

Although a variety of other models may be mixed in, or explicitly avowed, most psychiatric wards function primarily within a medical model. Doctors have final authority and decision making powers; medications are accorded primary therapeutic value and used extensively; the person is seen as having a disease, with attendant disability disfunction and dysfunction which is to be "treated" and "cured"; labeling and its consequences, objectification and stigmatization, are almost inevitable.

In contrast, at Soteria (from the Greek, salvation or deliverance) the primary focus is on growth, development and learning. The staff are to be with the patients, or residents as they are called, to facilitate these processes insofar as they can. They share decision-making powers and responsibility with residents. They are not there either to treat or cure the residents. Neuroleptic medications are infrequently used. Although we have no quarrel with the demonstrated heuristic value of the medical model, we believe its application to psychiatric disorders can have unfortunate (and unintended) consequences for individual patients. No alternative model is proposed, however, as none seem to satisfactorily explain what we label "schizophrenia." Our alternative stance is a phenomenologic approach to schizophrenia, an attempt to understand and share the psychotic person's experience without judging, labeling, derogating or invalidating it.

Size

Most psychiatric hospital wards have at least 20 patients. Thus, the staff/patient group is apt to be 40-60. For severely disorganized persons, however, a social reference group of no more than 12-15 persons is especially important. A group of this size, when combined with a homelike atmosphere, maximizes the possibility of the disorganized person's getting to know and trust a new environment and to find a surrogate family in it; at the same time, it minimizes the labeling and stigmatization process. This number is about the maximum number able to live under one roof as an extended family or commune. Most clinicians also believe 12 is about the upper limit for group therapy. Finally, experimental psychology's small task groups have been shown to function most effectively with not more than 12 members. Thus, rather than a 20-bed ward, Soteria is a home that sleeps 8-10 comfortably, with six beds occupied by residents and two by staff.

Social Structure

This aspect interacts closely with size. To function effectively, every organization, large or small, needs structure. In general, the larger the organization the greater the structure. Unfortunately, more elaborated structures have consequences which impinge negatively on persons undergoing psychotic disorganization: inflexibility, reliance on authority, institutionalization of roles and decision-making power residing in the hierarchy. These are outside the client's control. Inevitably, those at the bottom of the hierarchy feel powerless, irresponsible and dependent. Because of this, Soteria is as unstructured as is commensurate with adequate function. Structure which develops to meet functional needs is dissolved if the need is not a continuing one. There is no institutionalized method of dealing with a particular occurrence. For example, overt aggressive acts are dealt with in a variety of ways including physical control, depending on a myriad of contextual variables.

Medication

We live in an overmedicated, too frequently drug-dependent culture. Our ambivalence about drugs is resolved by creating two categories of drugs: good ones (e.g., alcohol) and bad ones (e.g., LSD). Psychiatry's attitude is no different from that of the wider social context; the magical answer is sought from a pill. The antipsychotic drugs have provided psychiatry with real substance for their magical cure fantasy with regard to schizophrenia. As is the case with most such exaggerated expectations, the fantasy is better than the reality. After 25 years, it is now clear that the antipsychotics do not *cure* schizophrenia. It is also clear that they have serious, sometimes irreversible toxicities (Crane, 1973), that recovery may be impaired by them in at least some schizophrenics (Goldstein, 1970; Rappaport, et al., 1978) and that they have little effect on long-term psychosocial adjustment (Niskanen and Achte, 1972). This is not to deny their extraordinary helpfulness in reducing and controlling symptoms, shortening hospital stays and revitalizing interest in schizophrenia. One aim of the Soteria project is to seek a viable, informed alternative to the overuse of, and excessive reliance on, these drugs–often to the exclusion of psychosocial measures. We use them infrequently and when prescribed, they are kept primarily under the patient's control. That is, the resident is asked to monitor his response to the drug carefully, to give us feedback so we can adjust dosage, and after a trial period of two weeks he is given a major voice in determining whether or not the drug will be continued.

Soteria is a reaction to criticisms of existing facilities in each of the four areas mentioned above. However, much of what is involved in the program is based on the positive contributions of a variety of other researchers, clinicians and theorists. In fact, we recognize that no individual element of the Soteria program is new; it is their combination in one setting we believe to be unique.

Some of Soteria's roots are the era of moral treatment in America (Bockoven, 1963), the tradition of intensive interpersonal intervention in schizophrenia (Sullivan, 1962; Fromm-Reichmann, 1948), therapists who have described growth from psychosis (Menninger, 1959; Perry, 1962), the group of psychiatric heretics (Laing, 1967; Szasz, 1961) and descriptions of the development of psychiatric disorder in response to life crisis (Brown and Birley, 1968).

Sample Selection

All subjects are obtained from a screening facility that is part of the CMHC complex containing our control wards. Approximately 600 new patients are seen there per month, of whom about 250 are hospitalized. Anyone meeting the following basic criteria is a potential study candidate:

1. Clearly schizophrenic
2. Deemed in need of hospitalization
3. No more than one previous hospitalization for 4 weeks or less with a diagnosis of schizophrenia
4. Age 18-30 (either sex)
5. Unmarried, separated, widowed or divorced.

The selection criteria are designed to provide a relatively homogeneous sample of individuals diagnosed schizophrenic, but a group at risk for prolonged hospitalization or chronic disability. Early onset and being unmarried have been shown to predict a need for chronic care (Strauss, et al., 1977).

Because of research grant related changes (see Treatment Assignments below) Soteria treated subjects are divided into two cohorts, 1971-76 and 1976-83. There are 37 experimental and 42 controls in the first and 20 experimental and 24 controls in the second cohort.

Treatment Assignments

Subjects meeting study selection criteria are identified without knowledge of the group to which they will ultimately be assigned. Study requirements are explained and informed consent is obtained from the patient and his family, or significant other, if available. In the 1971-76 study cohort, because of limited experimental bed availability, subjects were assigned on a consecutively admitted, space available basis. Subjects in the 1976-83 cohort were assigned on a strictly random basis.

Research Assessment

The measures below are a partial list of those completed at baseline (admission to the study) and at followup (6, 12 and 24 months postadmission). All assessments are conducted by an independent research team that has no direct treatment responsibilities in either setting.

Baseline

Diagnosis–As per diem DSM-II (American Psychiatric Association 1968). For a subject to be included in the study, three independent diagnoses of schizophrenia must be in agreement.

Diagnosis symptoms–A checklist of seven symptoms. Four of seven symptoms are required for inclusion in the study (Cole, Klerman, and Goldberg, 1964).

Certainty of diagnosis–A 7-point scale (Mosher, Pollin, and Stabenau, 1971).

Mode of onset–Assesses acute/insidious onset types (Vaillant, 1964).

Paranoid/nonparanoid status–A short scale for rating paranoid schizophrenia (Venables and O'Connor, 1959).

Global severity–An overall measure of psychopathology.

Brief Social History Form–A detailed description of a patient's and family's psychiatric and social history (Boothe, Schooler, and Goldberg, 1972).

Followup

Patient Progress Report–For each 6-month interval, information on the subject's medication history, use of other treatment, living arrangements (including any hospital readmissions), work status, social contacts, global severity and improvement is obtained.

CLINICAL SETTINGS

Experimental

Soteria is located on a busy street in a transitional neighborhood of a San Francisco Bay Area city. Bordering Soteria on one side is a nursing home and on the other, a two-family home. The neighborhood has a mixture of small businesses, medical facilities (a general hospital is one block away), single-family homes and small apartments (usually homes that have been remodeled for this purpose). It is a designated poverty area inhabited by a mixture of college students, lower-class families and ex-state hospital patients. Some 15-20 percent of residents in the area are Mexican-American and there is a sprinkling of blacks.

Due primarily to licensing laws, the house can accommodate only six residents at one time, although as many as ten persons can sleep there comfortably. There are six paid nonprofessional staff plus the house director and a 1/4 time project psychiatrist. One or two new residents are admitted each month. In general, two of our specially trained nonprofessional staff, a man and a woman, are on duty at any one time. In addition, there are usually one or more volunteers present, especially in the evening. Most staff work 36 to 48-hour shifts to provide themselves the opportunity to relate to "spaced-out" (their term) residents continuously over a relatively long period of time. Staff and residents share responsibility for household maintenance, meal preparation and cleanup. Persons who are not "together" are not expected to do an equal share of the work. Over the long term, staff do more than their share and will step in to assume responsibility if a resident cannot do a task to which he has agreed. The house director acts as friend, counselor, supervisor and object for displaced angry feelings by staff. The part-time project psychiatrist supervises the staff and is seen as a stable, reassuring presence in addition to his formal medico-legal responsibilities

Although staff vary in how they see their roles, they generally view what psychiatry labels a "schizophrenic reaction" as an altered state of consciousness in an individual who is experiencing a crisis in living. Simply put, the altered state involves personality fragmentation with the loss of a sense of self.

Few clinicians would disagree with a description of the evolution of psychosis as a process of fragmentation and disintegration. But, at Soteria House, the disruptive psychotic experience is also believed to have unique potential for reintegration and reconstitution if it is not prematurely aborted or forced into a psychologically straitjacketing compromise. This is in keeping with the ethos at Kingsley Hall. Such a view of schizophrenia implies a number of therapeutic attitudes. All facets of the psychotic experience are taken by staff members as "real." They view the experiential and behavioral attitudes associated with the psychosis—the clinical symptoms, including irrationality, terror and mystical experiences—as extremes of basic human qualities. Because "irrational" behavior and mystical beliefs are regarded as valid, Soteria staff try to provide an atmosphere that will facilitate integration of the psychosis into the continuity of the individual's life. Thus, psychotic persons are not to be considered "diseased," nor related to in a depersonalized way; to do so would invalidate the experience.

When the fragmentation process is seen as valid with potential for psychological growth, the individual experiencing the schizophrenic reaction is tolerated, lived with, related to and validated, but not "treated" or used to fulfill staff needs. Limits are set if the person is clearly a danger to himself, others or the program as a whole—not merely because others are unable to tolerate his madness. Antipsychotic drugs are ordinarily not used for more than six weeks. If the resident shows no change at that time and is either paranoid or has an insidious onset, neuroleptic drugs are instituted at appropriate dosage levels.

Why use trained nonprofessionals as primary staff (see also Mosher et al., 1973, and Hirschfeld et al., 1977)? Relatively untrained, psychologically unsophisticated persons can assume a phenomenological stance vis-a-vis psychosis more easily than highly trained persons (e.g., M.D.s or Ph.D.s) because they have learned no theory of schizophrenia, whether psychodynamic, organic or a combination of both.

Lacking the preconceived ideas of professionals, our nonprofessional staff can be themselves, follow their visceral responses and be a "person" with the psychotic individual. Highly trained mental health professionals tend to lose this freedom in favor of a more cognitive, theory-based, learned response that may invalidate a patient's experience of himself if the professional's theory-based behavior is not congruent with the patient's felt needs. Professionals may also use their theoretical knowledge defensively when confronted in an unstructured setting, with anxiety-provoking behaviors of psychotic persons. This pattern of response is not so readily available to our unsophisticated nonprofessional therapists, nor is it reinforced by a professional degree with its accompanying status and power.

CMHC Comparison Ward

The Community Mental Health Center's inpatient service consists of two locked wards of 30 beds each. About 250 patients are admitted (including readmissions) per month. It is a well-staffed (1.5/1 staff/patient ratio) active treatment facility oriented towards crisis intervention, employing high doses of neuroleptics, rapid evaluation and placement in other parts of the county's treatment network as its immediate goal. All of the control patients reported here received antipsychotic drugs during their inpatient stays. Only one was discharged off drugs.

The CMHC staff is generally well trained, experienced and enthusiastic; they see themselves as doing a good job. Patients are assigned to one of five treatment teams on each ward which meet daily to decide treatment plans. The assigned therapist provides one-half hour of psychotherapy daily and takes a major role in treatment planning. The therapist may be a technician, community worker or any of the other treatment specialists. There are 1-1/2 hours per day of occupational therapy and a daily community meeting led by any member of the treatment team. A crisis group meets for 1-1/2 hours five times per week (all patients); a couples group, two hours per week (married patients and spouses); a psychodrama group, two hours per week (all patients who are able); a women's group, two hours per week; and a survival group 1-1/2 hours (for readmitted patients) three times each week.

Because the Center inpatient service takes patients from all over the county (it is the only facility with a 24-hour-a-day psychiatric emergency service and locked wards), most patients are referred back to one of four regional centers nearest their homes for outpatient care. This care may include partial hospitalization (day or night care), individual, family or group therapy and medication followup. The county also has an extensive board and care system and eight halfway houses for adolescents and adults.

Although the present report focuses only on Soteria House and its hospital comparison ward, a second experimental facility, Emanon House, was established in a nearby county in 1974. It is compared with its own nearby general hospital psychiatric ward. The research design is the same for both project facilities.

RESULTS

Six week outcome data for all Soteria House subjects and two-year outcome data from the subjects admitted between 1971 and 76 have been reported in detail elsewhere (Mosher and Menn, 1978; Matthews et al., 1979; Mosher et al., 1989). Briefly summarized, the significant results are:

1. Admission characteristics: Subjects in the two programs are remarkably similar on most demographic and admission psychiatric variables.

2. Six week outcome: In terms of psychopathology, subjects in both groups improved significantly and comparably, despite Soteria subjects having not received neuroleptic.

3. Milieu assessments: Because Soteria programs is a recovery-facility social environment, systematic study and comparison of the two milieus are particularly important. We have used Moos' WAS and COPES scale for this purpose (Moos, 1974). The between-program differences, we find, have been remarkable in their magnitude and stability over ten years. As may be seen in Figure 1, the Soteria environment is perceived as significantly different from the CMHC milieu on 9 of 10 subscales of the Moos

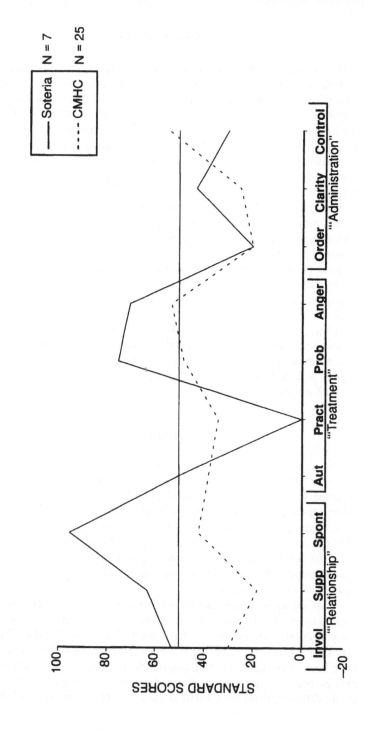

FIGURE 1. Comparison of Soteria Staff and CMHC Staff WAS Real Testing Based on Staff Norms for 160 Wards

instrument. They are similar on only the order and organization variable. This pattern has remained stable with minor fluctuations for the project's 10-year life. Thus we conclude that the two environments are, in fact, very different with Soteria milieu, conforming closely to our predictions (Wendt et al., 1983).

4. Community psychosocial adjustment: At two years postadmission, Soteria-treated subjects from the 1971-76 cohort were working at significantly higher occupational levels and were more often living independently or with peers. These data from the 1976-83 cohort are not yet available.

5. In the first cohort, despite the large differences in lengths of stay during the initial admissions (about one versus five months), the cost of the first 6 months of care for both groups is about $4,000.

SYSTEM CHANGE

To summarize, the Soteria project suggests that newly diagnosed schizophrenic patients can be treated as well–or better–at no greater cost in a nonhospital community setting as a hospital. Our results are consistent with those of others who studied nonhospital alternative treatments, e.g., Fairweather et al., 1969; Pasamanick, 1967; Stein and Test, 1976; Langsley et al., 1968; Polak and Kirby, 1976. Straw (1982) found that in 19 of 20 studies the outcomes were as good or better in the alternative treated groups when compared with those receiving hospital care. Has this scientific evidence resulted in a shift away from hospitals to use of alternative methods of care in the United States? Basically, the answer is no.

The evidence has not persuaded private psychiatry in the USA that non-hospital alternatives are useful. As indicated in the Laing memoir just preceding, this is no longer true in American public mental health where the notion of "Crisis Residences" has caught on (see Stroul, 1987).

Why, in the era of so-called "scientific" psychiatry, have these types of facilities and clinical care paradigms not been widely implemented?

The most facile answers are that the studies were insufficiently rigorous, did not provide convincing evidence or were one-time, unreplicable products of the investigators' enthusiasm and dedication. As one of these enthusiastic investigators, I must ask how many comparative outcome studies of variations in hospital treatment are there? Despite the more than a million patients psychiatrically hospitalized each year in the U.S., there are very few controlled outcome studies of systematically varied inpatient care (Glick et al., 1974; Herz et al., 1971; Caffey et al., 1972). While the evidence supporting alternatives may not be incontrovertible, there would appear to be more hard data relative to their usefulness than there are for in-hospital treatment.

If the evidence presented is acceptable, why is the next step—its application to clinical care settings—not? I would posit that the implementation of alternatives is unacceptable because they represent a threat to in-hospital psychiatry's turf. What are the elements of the Soteria program (these are true to a greater or lesser extent for most alternatives) perceived as threats to hospital psychiatry?

In brief, the elements of the Soteria program most relevant to this discussion are:

1. The facility is not a hospital and its program is not run by doctors or nurses by delegation. However, it admits only clients who would have otherwise been hospitalized.
2. Neuroleptics, the standard treatment for schizophrenia, are used as infrequently as possible, preferably not at all.
3. Primary treatment responsibility, power and authority are vested in the nonprofessional staff.

How has traditional hospital psychiatry defended itself against this rather radical attempt to demedicalize psychosis? We will describe four that we believe to be most used to maintain the *status quo*.

1. Foremost, and most effective, there are no third-party payers in the U.S. willing to underwrite this form of care. Psychiatry has not actively moved to prevent third-party payment for alternatives, but it has not actively sought it.

The ultimate viability of alternatives in the therapeutic market place resides with funding sources—which is why they are becoming available in public systems but not in private ones. The degree of interest these fiscal intermediaries will have in paying for innovations in care is strongly influenced by the prevailing zeitgeist. In the last decade or so there has been a substantial shift in American psychiatry's zeitgeist away from a socio-environmental one to a more medical biologic point of view. Thus, there is little pressure from biomedically oriented mainstream psychiatry to pay for a basically nonmedical treatment. What are other relevant manifestations of the biomedical zeitgeist? It would appear that psychiatry is doing what it believes it must to continue to qualify for third-party payment, i.e., sticking with hospital-based wards.

2. The medicalization of community psychiatry. It is ironic that the now nearly 30-year-old community psychiatry movement in the U.S. has moved the mental health system back into closer juxtaposition with the somatic health system. That is, the relative isolation of mental health

before the 1960s—as manifested in the state hospital systems—was broken down with the advent of community psychiatry with its emphasis on inpatient care on wards in general medical hospitals. The growth of such wards was also given impetus by psychiatric coverage in various health insurance programs and by government sponsored medicare and medicaid. For the most part, payment for inpatient care in general hospitals has been the only consistently available mental health benefit. These two factors account in large part for growth of these wards and the increasing numbers of patients treated in them. For example, between 1967 and 1971, the numbers of schizophrenic patients treated on such wards nearly doubled—from 90,000 to 170,000 (Taube, 1969, 1973).

This process of bringing "mental illness" back into the mainstream of medicine was given further impetus by a flurry of developments in medical technology. That is, a whole array of new, sophisticated techniques became available for use in the search for the "schizococcus" and other specific etiologies of mental illness. Application of these techniques to "mental illness" has provided us with a deluge of new information but has as yet failed to discover specific etiologic factors in psychosis. In a characteristically American fashion, a new generation of technology-oriented biological psychiatrists has risen preferentially to positions of influence and power in many medical school departments of psychiatry.

3. Neuroleptics. Another important factor in the progressive medicalization of madness has been the introduction and widespread use of neuroleptic drugs—clearly efficacious treatments for psychosis. Because drugs can only be prescribed by M.D.s, as long as drugs are viewed as "the answer" to mental illness, doctors' power and control of the treatment system are inevitable and will increase.

Because pills are given to individuals, they maintain medicine's traditional focus on *a* person as "sick." This can prevent the doctor and the system over which he presides from looking at the family and wider social contextual factors that might have exerted important influences on the development of psychosis and might also therefore be amenable to intervention. Thus, medications can narrow conceptual sights and unnecessarily limit treatment possibilities.

4. The waning influence of psychoanalysis. It is fair to say that the '50s and early '60s were the heyday of psychoanalytic influence on more traditional psychiatry. Psychoanalysts and analytic theories were widely used for both descriptive and etiologic purposes. For a number of years, residents in the best known training programs entered analytic training.

In the late '60s and through the '70s their influence has been much diluted by waves of findings from the new technologists and technology.

The appeal of analytic constructs, so pervasive in the '50s and '60s, has been replaced by more reliably identifiable and quantifiable neurotransmitters, endorphins, etc. Whether these high-tech findings have made a substantial contribution to clinical practice remains moot.

This evolution is complex, but psychoanalysis is not as interested in psychosis as it was during its halcyon days. The neuroleptics, development of rapid turnover wards in general hospitals and community psychiatry each contributed to what I perceive as a withdrawal of psychoanalysis' cathexis of psychosis. It seems to have given up psychosis in favor of a return to the original turf of analysis—the outpatient treatment of neurosis.

This brief discussion is obviously oversimplified, biased and subject to many exceptions. However, it does give one person's perception—with little vested interest in the process—of a facet of recent history.

CONCLUSION

The Soteria project closed its data collection and treatment facility in 1983 but data analysis has continued. What have we learned so far from the second generation Kingsley Hall?

1. It is possible to establish and maintain an interpersonally based therapeutic milieu that is as effective as neuroleptic in reducing the acute symptoms of psychosis in the short term (six weeks) in *newly diagnosed psychotics*.

2. The therapeutic community personnel do not require extensive mental health training and experience to be effective in the experimental context. They do, however, need to be sure that this is the type of work they want to do, be psychologically strong, tolerant and flexible, and positive and enthusiastic. Finally, they need good on-the-job training and easily accessible supervision and backup.

3. Longer term outcomes (two years) for the Soteria treated group are as good or better than those of the hospital treated control subjects in terms of independence, autonomy and peer based social networks. In addition, more than 80% of the experimental group have little or no risk of tardive dyskinesia as they received little or no antipsychotic drug treatment over the followup period.

4. Although it is difficult to confirm or dismiss from the data it appears that the positive longer term outcomes achieved by the Soteria treated subjects are at least in part due to the spontaneous growth of a Soteria-related, easily accessible, social network around the facility. It provides interpersonal support, housing, jobs, friends and recreational activities as needed to ex-Soteria clients and staff.

REFERENCES

Bockoven J: *Moral Treatment in American Psychiatry.* New York: Springer Publishing Co. (1963).

Boothe H, Schooler N, Goldberg S: Brief social history for studies in schizophrenia: an announcement of a new data collection instrument. *Psychopharmacology Bulletin* 8:23-44, 1972.

Brown GW, Birley JLT: Crisis and life changes and the onset of schizophrenia. *J Health and Social Behav* 9:203-214, 1968.

Caffey EM, Galbrecht CR, Klett CJ: Brief hospitalization and aftercare in the treatment of schizophrenia. *Archives of General Psychiatry* 24:81-86, 1972.

Cole J, Klerman G, Goldberg S: Effectiveness of phenothiazine treatment in acute schizophrenics. *Archives of General Psychiatry* 10:246-261, 1964.

Crane G: Clinical psychopharmacology in its 20th year. *Science* 181:124-128, 1973.

Fairweather G, Sanders D, Cressler D, Maynard H: *Community Life for the Mentally Ill: An Alternative to Institutional Care.* Chicago: Adline Publishing Co. (1969).

Fromm-Reichmann F: Notes on the development of treatment of schizophrenia by psychoanalytic psychotherapy. *Psychiatry* 11:263-273, 1948.

Glick I, Hargreaves WA, Goldfield MD: Short vs. long hospitalization: a controlled prospective study. *Archives of General Psychiatry* 30:363-369, 1974.

Goldstein M: Premorbid adjustment, paranoid status, and patterns of response to phenothiazine in acute schizophrenia. *Schizophrenia Bulletin* 3:24-37, 1970.

Herz MI, Endicott J, Spitzer R, Mesnikoff A: Day vs. inpatient hospitalization. *American Journal of Psychiatry* 127(10):107-118, 1971.

Hirschfeld R, Matthews S, Mosher LR, Menn AZ: Being with madness: personality characteristics of three treatment staffs. *Hospital and Community Psychiatry* 28(4):267-273, 1977.

Klerman G, DiMascio A, Weissman M, Prusoff B, Paykel ES: Treatment of depression by drugs and psychotherapy. *American Journal of Psychiatry* 131:186-191, 1974.

Laing R: *The Politics of Experience.* New York: Ballantine Books (1967).

Langsley DG, Kaplan DM, Pittman FS, Machotka P, Flomenhaft K, DeYoung CD: *The Treatment of Families in Crisis.* New York: Grune and Stratton (1968).

Matthews SM, Roper MT, Mosher LR, Menn AZ: A non-neuroleptic treatment for schizophrenia: analysis of the two-year postdischarge risk of relapse. *Schizophrenia Bulletin* 5(2):322-333, 1979.

Menninger K: *Psychiatrist's World: The Selected Papers of Karl Menninger.* Edited by B. Hall. New York: Viking Press (1959).

Moos RH: *Evaluating Treatment Environments: A Social Ecological Approach.* New York: John Wiley and Sons (1974).

Mosher L, Pollin W, Stabenau J: Identical twins discordant for schizophrenia: neurologic findings. *Archives of General Psychiatry* 24:422-430, 1971.

Mosher L, Reifman A, Menn A: Characteristics of nonprofessionals serving as primary therapists for acute schizophrenics. *Hospital and Community Psychiatry* 24:391-395, 1973.

Mosher LR, Menn A: Community residential treatment for schizophrenia: two-year followup data. *Hospital & Community Psychiatry* 29:715-723, 1978.

Mosher LR, Vallone R, Menn AZ: The soteria project: new outcome data ("il progetto soteria: nuovi resultati emersi"). In A. Migone, G. Martini and V. Volterra (Eds), *New Trends In Schizophrenia*. Caserta: Edito dalla Fondazione, pp. 313-330, 1989.

Niskanen P, Achte K: *The Course and Prognosis of Schizophrenic Psychoses in Helsinki: A Comparative Study of First Admissions in 1950.* Monograph No. 2 from the Psychiatric Clinic of the Helsinki University Central Hospital, 1972.

Pasamanick B, Scarpitti FD, Dinitz S: *Schizophrenics In the Community.* New York: Appleton-Century-Crofts (1967).

Perry J: Reconstitutive process in the psychopathology of the self. *Annals of the New York Academy of Sciences* 96:853-876, 1962.

Polak PR, Kirby MW: A model to replace psychiatric hospitals. *J Nerv Ment Dis* 162:13-22, 1976.

Rappaport M, Hopkins HK, Hall K, Belleza T, Silverman J: Are there schizophrenics for whom drugs may be unnecessary or contraindicated? *International Pharmacopsychiatry* 13:100-111, 1978.

Stein LI, Test MA: Training in community living: One year evaluation. *Am J Psychiatry* 133:917-918, 1976.

Strauss JS, Kokes RF, Klorman R, Sacksteder JL: Premorbid adjustment in schizophrenia: concepts, measures, and implications. Part I. The concept of premorbid adjustment. *Schizophrenia Bulletin* 3(2) 182-185, 1977.

Straw RB: Meta-analysis of deinstitutionalization. Ann Arbor, Mich.: Northwestern University (1982). Doctoral dissertation.

Stroul BA: *Crisis Residential Services In a Community Support System.* Report to the NIMH Community Support Program. Rockville, MD (1987).

Sullivan H: *Schizophrenia As a Human Process.* New York: W. W. Norton and Co. (1962).

Szasz T: *The Myth of Mental Illness: Foundations of a Theory of a Personal Conduct.* New York: Hoeber-Harper (1961).

Taube C: *Length of Stay of Discharges from General Hospital Psychiatric Inpatient Units. United States 1970-1971.* Statistical Note 70. Biometry Branch, NIMH, 1973.

Taube C: *General Hospital Inpatient Psychiatric Services 1967.* Survey and Reports Section, Biometry Branch, Office of Program Planning and Evaluation, NIMH, 1969.

Vaillant G: Prospective prediction of schizophrenic remission. *Archives of General Psychiatry* 11:509-515, 1964.

Venables P, O'Connor N: A short scale for rating paranoid schizophrenia. *Journal of Mental Science* 105:815-818, 1959.

Wendt J, Mosher LR, Matthews S, Menn A: A comparison of two treatment environments for schizophrenia. In: Gunderson JG, Will OA, Jr., Mosher LR, eds. *Psychiatric Milieu and the Therapeutic Process.* New York: Jason Aronson, Inc., pp. 17-33, 1983.

Perceptions of Psychologists
and Psychiatrists

Victor D. Sanua

SUMMARY. The purpose of this paper is to review surveys that have been conducted to evaluate the perceptions of the general public towards psychologists and psychiatrists. There are two major studies, one in Canada and the other in Atlanta, Georgia commissioned by psychiatry. Only minor studies have been conducted by psychologists. There seems to be a consistent finding that psychologists rate very well among the general public, while psychiatrists seem to have an image problem. There has been a decided decrease of physicians going into psychiatry, while the field of psychology is thriving and the number of psychological associations is increasing. In the Canadian study, it was revealed that about 75% of respondents are hesitant to see a psychiatrist because they "are too ready to prescribe drugs." In the Atlanta survey, 83% of the respondents indicated that they would feel uncomfortable seeing a psychiatrist. In one research, a group of individuals were least satisfied with their contacts with psychiatrists who dealt primarily with the medication of a sick relative.

These findings are of extreme importance in view of the efforts of a large number of clinical psychologists who would like to have prescription privileges. It is felt that on the basis of these findings, psychologists should have a better evaluation of their own profession. We can do better than psychiatrists! *[Article copies available from The Haworth Document Delivery Service: 1-800-342-9678.]*

Victor D. Sanua, PhD, is affiliated with the Department of Psychology, St. John's University, Jamaica, NY 11439.

[Haworth co-indexing entry note]: "Perceptions of Psychologists and Psychiatrists." Sanua, Victor D. Co-published simultaneously in *The Psychotherapy Patient* (The Haworth Press, Inc.) Vol. 9, No. 3/4, 1996, pp. 59-75; and: *Psychosocial Approaches to Deeply Disturbed Persons* (eds: Peter R. Breggin, and E. Mark Stern) The Haworth Press, Inc., 1996, pp. 59-75. Single or multiple copies of this article are available from The Haworth Document Delivery Service [1-800-342-9678, 9:00 a.m. - 5:00 p.m. (EST)].

At this time of the rapid development of the profession of psychology and the continual efforts on the part of psychiatry to limit the professional legitimacy of psychology as a provider of mental health services and reduce the standing of our field, particularly with their powerful lobby in Washington, D.C., it behooves us to get an overview of the feelings and the attitude of the general public towards these professions. It is also useful to examine how other mental health professionals view psychology. For the longest period of time and still to some extent today, there seems to be confusion about the functions of these two professions. One outstanding difference known by the majority of the educated public is that psychiatrists have an M.D. degree and can prescribe drugs while psychologists have a Ph.D. degree but cannot prescribe drugs.

The purpose of this paper is to evaluate the image that the general public has of psychology and psychiatry, how psychiatrists and psychologists view each other. The data available which would provide information on each aspect of the question tend to be rather scarce. It is somewhat surprising that in spite of the research orientation of psychologists, they have not pursued research to "know themselves" better through an analysis of the attitudes of the general public towards the profession. Rosario Webb and Ramsay Speer (1986) have pointed out that research on this issue is meager, dated, and of questionable methodology.

To get some idea about the differences in public's attitude towards psychiatry and psychology, we have to refer to two studies conducted by two market research organizations commissioned and financed by the psychiatric establishment. One study was conducted in Ontario, Canada, and the other in the U.S.A. We have not been able to locate an adequate study by psychologists regarding the general public's attitude towards psychiatry and psychology. This is somewhat surprising because there is a feeling that psychologists are not receiving adequate respect from the general public, or possibly that the same public has a more favorable picture of psychiatrists, particularly in view of their medical degree. Is it possible that psychologists suffer from some inferiority feelings? As the paper develops, data will reveal that such feelings are misplaced. Naturally, one of the criteria for such low self-evaluation is that psychiatrists make more money than psychologists. I recall a discussion I had with a psychiatrist when I told him that APA stands for the American Psychological Association, while ApA (small p) stands for the American Psychiatric Association because of the much larger number of trained psychologists than psychiatrists in the U.S.A. His immediate answer was that this was true, but the fact remains that they still make more money, a fact that cannot be denied.

In 1988, the Ontario Psychiatric Association (O.P.A.) commissioned the organization Cormark Communications Inc. to conduct research into the attitudes of the Ontario public towards psychiatry in view of O.P.A.'s plan to introduce a public relations campaign directed towards the Ontario general public ("Canadian survey," 1989). Fortunately the study included a number of questions about psychology. The following is a summary of the report.

In terms of perceived effectiveness, the majority (54% of 751) responses on the mailed questionnaires indicated that the competence of psychiatrists and psychologists was about equal in helping people overcome their problems. The remaining respondents were about equally split: half felt that psychiatrists were more effective, while the other half chose psychologists as being more effective. Thus on the basis of this finding, it seems that the M.D. degree does not give an aura of superiority to the profession of psychiatry, at least in Ontario. Respondents were provided a number of reasons for hesitating to see a psychiatrist. The issue which generated the greatest concern was the possibility that a psychiatrist might be "too ready to prescribe drugs" as part of the treatment. The total percentage of those who were hesitant to go to a psychiatrist because of the possibility of having drugs prescribed, was 77% (23% indicated great concern; 32% some concern; and 22% expressed slight concern). This certainly comes as a revelation, also supported by further research to be discussed in this paper, at this time when there are strong influences within the APA which consider prescription privileges as representing a normal evolutionary development in the expansion of the profession of psychology or "a logical evolution of professional practice" (DeLeon, Folen, Jennings, Willis & al (1991). Only 15% of the respondents agreed with the statement: "Psychiatrists are generally well balanced people who have their lives in control," 40% disagreed; and 45% were unwilling to state how they felt one way or another. Insofar as respect is concerned, 4 out of 10 responded that psychiatrists were less respected than other medical doctors, four indicated that they were respected to the same extent; and only 1 out of 10 felt that psychiatrists commanded more respect than other medical doctors. On the basis of these findings, Edward Waring, former president of the Canadian Psychiatric Association, indicated that "obviously, there is a lot of opportunity for public education" (p. 14).

Since 1987, The Keckley Group of Atlanta, Georgia ("Psychiatry: Fact and Perceptions," 1991) has been conducting studies on psychiatry in 10 markets representing a cross-section of opinion and geography. I shall only include here the data as it pertains to the comparison between psychiatrists and psychologists. Approximately 56% of psychologists agree that "psychiatrists treat psychology unfairly. They take advantage of the system, and they don't treat us as equals." Furthermore, 39% felt that "psychiatrists don't understand psychologists, as they don't ask our opinion." Three quarters of benefit managers noted that they were "considering changes in the way health benefits were provided for these types of problems." Naturally this reflects the increasing pressure placed on businesses by spiraling mental-health-care costs. While 72% of consumers agreed that "psychiatry is necessary–all of us need help sometimes," 83% said they would feel "uncomfortable seeing a psychiatrist." Sixty-two percent said they would "rather see a psychologist than a psychiatrist." While 53% of the consumers were able to identify in relevant terms psychiatrists, 43% were able to do so for psychologists, a disparity which might not be meaningful in spite of the fact that a significant difference for many is that the psychiatrist is an M.D. Using a scale of 1 to 10 (with 10 being the highest mark), consumers were asked to score a variety of health professionals on their academic training and competence. While the rating for psychiatrists was 5.1, for clinical psychologists it was 4.8. As in the previous report, psychologists appear to fare rather well. It would seem from the Keckley's study that psychiatry in general is not viewed more favorably in comparison to psychology.

Recent data show that psychiatry as a profession has tended to decline in view of the smaller number of new physicians going into the field of psychiatry. A recent article in the *Psychiatric News* (Cody, 1993) indicates that psychiatry has had a difficult time getting physicians to specialize in psychiatry. In 1988, 746 were recruited. In 1993, only 477 were going into the profession, and this is happening at a time when available residencies are increasing. Only three states filled their psychiatric residency positions: New Hampshire, Vermont and Utah.

This decline of psychiatry was confirmed by a column of APA president Frank Farley when he wrote in the APA *Monitor,* July, 1993 that "Psychiatry appears to be declining in membership. . . . Social work thrives, but continues primarily to be a non-doctoral field. A great strength of psychology lies in its inclusion of both science and practice in the same discipline. Serious problems have arisen in other fields where practice was divorced from science" (p. 3).

The fact that psychiatrists have little regard for psychologists is confirmed by various statements made recently by the leadership of the American Psychiatric Association. I shall provide only a few quotations reflecting their attitudes, particularly in connection with the training of psychologists as mental health workers, at least in their public pronouncement. Fink, a former President of the American Psychiatric Association, wrote the following:

> Psychologists and other non-psychiatrists "don't have the training to make the initial evaluation and diagnosis" and "are not trained to understand the nuances of the mind. . . . Doctors should refer to doctors." (*American Medical News,* Feb. 12, 1988, quotations are found in Wright and Spielberger, 1989)

Sabshin, Medical Director of ApA, in addressing psychiatrists in general, writes the following in the Newsletter of the Pennsylvania Psychiatric Association (Dec. 1988-Jan. 1989):

> . . . physicians in every state must meet continuing education requirements, yet psychologists have continuing education requirements in fewer than 15 states. If psychologists wish to practice medicine, their medical degrees ought to be conferred by medical schools, not state legislatures or regulatory agencies. Furthermore, psychologists should not be able to hide behind the simplistic and erroneous claim that they provide services analogous to health care by psychiatrists, but at significant cost-saving to their clients. . . . While recognizing that psychologists have a role to play in our health care system, I urge legislative scrutiny of their attempts to be that which they are not. In doing so, we physicians affirm our professional commitment to quality health care. (Reported by Wright and Spielberger, 1989)

According to Wright and Spielberger, the truth about continuing education is that for physicians' re-licensure it is needed in 22 states compared to 19 for psychologists. For a more adequate review of the efforts of the psychiatric establishment to prevent psychologists from providing mental health services because of their supposed incompetence to deal with "medical mental illness," the reader is referred to a review by Sanua (1993).

As a counter argument to the above statements made by psychiatrists that psychologists are not competent to diagnose mental disorders or formulate treatment plans and that patients may be harmed if treated by psychotherapy without the supervision of a psychiatrist, Dörken (1990) reviewed 13 years of professional liability of psychologists and showed that there has never been a court award against any insured psychologist for failure to refer to a physician when needed. This certainly weakens the argument by the above two leading psychiatrists that psychologists are not adequate to the task of providing mental health care. It is to be noted that psychiatric malpractice insurance costs 3-24 times more than psychological malpractice. Of course, this is because the administration of drugs entails risks to patients. The following quotation by Dörken explains the problem of using organic approaches in the treatment of mental disorders:

> The high-risk assaultive procedures pioneered by psychiatry of deep insulin coma therapy, prefrontal lobotomy, and regressive shock are now ventures of the past based largely on conjecture. . . . Thus the clear major difference between psychiatric and psychological practice is the capacity of psychiatrists to prescribe drugs. (p. 151)

He points out that many patients kept under continued medication for too long have suffered permanent neurological impairment. For a detailed description of those risks the reader is referred to a review of the literature by Sanua (1990, 1993a).

The negative attitude towards psychology is not shared by a number of psychiatrists. Dietch, director of medical-student education in psychiatry at the University of California, wrote a letter to the Supreme Court in support of psychology. He stated that there is no research to show that patients treated by psychologists fare worse than those treated by psychiatrists, who, on the other hand, may harm patients by improperly prescribing psychotropic drugs (Buie, 1988).

According to psychiatrists Webb and Edward (1982), psychiatrists are not well trained either in psychology or medicine. They write:

> Their [psychiatrists'] dynamic formulations and vague references to systems theory are pale by comparison to [those of] well-trained experimental psychologists who know how to handle data, are knowledgeable about group process, and know how to be persuasive. Most of what modern psychologists know is well worth psychiatry's knowing. (p. 81)

He declares that psychologists armed with computers and paper and pencil tests offer a far more tempting "certainty" than the conceptual generalities offered by psychiatrists. Warner (1979) found that psychiatrists were almost twice as likely to diagnose psychosis than other mental health professionals. One of the possible explanations is that psychiatrists could be motivated to diagnose psychosis more often, since it enables them to take a more active role in prescribing medication.

Regarding the training of the psychiatrist, I shall refer to two psychiatrists who, prior to their medical training had obtained a Ph.D. degree. Orne (1980), M.D. with a Ph.D. in clinical psychology, raises the serious question as to whether psychiatrists should be medically trained, as he delineates some of the problems of medical training. He argues that with such a background, the psychiatrist will focus on locating the diseases of the body that cause the problem, rather than searching for an appropriate appreciation of psychological causation. Thus, medical training could be counterproductive. He feels that a psychiatrist's skill demands experience in interpersonal relationships and an appreciation of the nuances of psychological causality. Fink, as noted earlier, stated that psychologists are not trained to know the "nuances of the mind" (see p. 5). The training of a psychiatrist starts immediately after his medical training. The internship had been eliminated, but it seems now to have become a requirement. The most significant aspect of the training is the day-to-day care the psychiatrist gives to patients and the formal and informal supervision he/she receives. Psychiatrists acquire skills on the job, and it is possible for them to become psychiatrists without having had a single course in psychology, sociology or anthropology. Thus they may lack the intellectual tools developed by the social sciences which could help resolve the kind of issues that should concern the profession.

Kingsbury (1987), who like Orne trained both as a psychologist and a psychiatrist, indicates that the psychologist is often lectured on the importance of the scientific approach and that knowledge is accumulated through sound methodology that would lead to replicability. Theories that enjoy some vogue can thus be easily discarded. The message the student gets is that while the scientific method always predominates and endures, theories do not. Students are also taught to read carefully the specifics of the sample selected and the validity and reliability of the tests used and to make sure that there are no extraneous factors that may affect the results. In contrast, in medical school the student is taught that science is a body of knowledge and procedures shared by those educated in the science. However, there are so many facts that develop that it would be difficult to master them; as a result, medical students depend on reviews with little space devoted to the manner in which the data were collected. The psychologist would be inclined to give a series of lectures to "introduce" a topic, while the physician would devote his lecture to discussing a "topic" in detail. While psychologists seem to be more inclined to reinforce their ideas by using references, psychiatrists are more apt to use clinical examples mostly from their own experience, e.g., "I've had good success using sedating phenothiazines to help manic patients" (Kingsbury, p. 155). Kingsbury states that the scientific base of psychiatry regarding the treatment of troubled people has increased very little in the last 20 years.

The following three studies consisted in asking various mental health professionals their views of their colleagues and on their own profession. Neimeyer & Walling (1990) asked groups of clinical psychologists, counseling psychologists, psychiatrists and social workers to rate their own and each of the other groups along three variables: attractiveness, expertise and trustworthiness. Results indicated that counseling psychologists and social workers were viewed as more attractive but less expert than clinical psychologists and psychiatrists. Clinical psychologists, counseling psychologists, and social workers were viewed as more trustworthy than psychiatrists. As expected, in no instance did any professional group rate another as significantly more attractive, trustworthy, or expert than itself, thus suggesting the operation of an in-group/out-group bias. Thus while psychologists were considered less attractive than counseling psychologists and social workers, they were considered to have more expertise, a quality shared by psychiatrists, but on the other hand, clinical psychologists were rated first in trustworthiness while psychiatrists were shown to be least trustworthy.

Janik and Kubickova (1990) asked specialists of five medical disciplines, a total of 360 specialists, to define the social prestige of their specialty. The sequence is as follows: surgeons, specialists in internal medicine, pediatricians, gynecologists and, in the last place, psychiatrists. The authors attribute the negative evaluation of psychiatry to its association with control and repressive functions performed by this discipline.

Koeske, Koeske and Mallinger (1993) examined the perception of self versus other among 101 professionals (social workers, psychologists and psychiatrists) regarding their effectiveness in intervention for 6 hypothetical clients representing a range of mental health problems. Psychiatrists were perceived as significantly less warm than social workers, even by psychiatrists themselves. For ratings of perceived expertise, an in-group preference was exhibited by psychologists and psychiatrists.

I shall now refer to a number of studies which have been conducted on a smaller scale than those mentioned earlier in this paper, in which a number of individuals belonging to specific groups were asked about their perception of psychologists, psychiatrists and other mental health workers. Alperin and Benedict (1985) reported that while psychiatrists were viewed by a group of college students, as "smart," they were also seen as "cold and reserved." Social workers were found to be warm but not particularly smart. Psychologists were not negatively stereotyped, and they were more likely to be consulted about personal problems.

Rosario Webb and Ramsay Speer (1986) administered a questionnaire to college students, (nonpsychology majors) and their parents. The authors wanted to discover what image they had about psychologists, psychiatrists, physicians, counselors, teachers and scientists. The results do not support the allegations of an unfavorable image of psychology. Rather they showed a favorable attitude towards psychologists, who were seen as very similar to psychiatrists and dissimilar to scientists. It was felt that the subjects' familiarity with psychologists was doubtful. However, Rosario Webb and Ramsay Speer believe that their study may mitigate psychologists' concerns about the public's perception of psychology. Rosario Webb (1989) in a later paper felt that a cross-section of the American public as represented by a Harris or Gallup poll would be of importance.

The next three studies refer to recent research on the public image of psychology. Only the most recent ones will be presented here, since we assume that more familiarity with the profession of psychology in recent years would result in more valid generalizations. In 1986 Wood, Jones and Benjamin provided a survey of the research on the public's image of psychology. Older surveys found that respondents could not differentiate between psychology and psychiatry, while later surveys revealed that the public is able to distinguish between the two professions. Former studies tended to view psychologists as more likely to be behavioral scientists and psychiatrists as more likely to be practitioners. Wood, Jones and Benjamin (1986) pointed out that recent studies on public opinion about psychologists relied on samples which were not representative of the current U.S.A. population. Carrying out their own research with 201 persons from four metropolitan areas: Los Angeles, Milwaukee, Houston, and Washington, D.C., they found that 84.43% agreed strongly or agreed somewhat that psychology is a science. They were asked to indicate which activities were more likely to be performed by psychologists and psychiatrists. They found that a large percentage of the sample believed psychologists rather than psychiatrists surveyed attitudes, predicted behavior and evaluated children in schools. Psychiatrists were found to be more likely (80.60% vs. 15.42%) to prescribe drugs. Respondents also demonstrated a moderate level of accuracy in their knowledge of the degree required to be a psychologist. About 40% indicated that they needed a Ph.D. degree. When respondents were asked about psychology's impact on their daily lives, 45.41% reported that it had an impact, and 81.32% were able to indicate the specific effect they had experienced. Because the most frequently mentioned type of impact on the respondents' daily lives concerned therapy, the most salient effect of psychology apparently includes mental health services. In conclusion, Wood, Jones and Benjamin (1986) believed that a fuller understanding of the public image of psychology can suggest ways in which organized psychology might better educate the public about the nature of its functions and significance for everyday life.

Schindler, Berren, Hannah, Beigel et al. (1987) administered a questionnaire to 119 patients at two community mental health centers and to 114 nonpatients to examine the public image of psychologists, psychiatrists, physicians and members of the clergy. The purpose was to evaluate the competence of various mental health workers on 10 specific types of patients. Psychiatrists were found to be more competent to deal with an alcoholic housewife, a sexually abused person and a paranoid man. Psychologists were found to be more competent to deal with a young couple, a teenage drug user, a disinterested couple and a lonely student; that is they were more effective in dealing with problems of adjustment and relationships. Neither was found to be more competent than the other in dealing with the following problems: a suicidal man, a depressed woman and an overactive child. As to the personal qualities exhibited by these two professionals, psychologists were found to be "warmer," and "more caring" than psychiatrists, while psychiatrists were found to have "more education and experience in mental health than psychologists." Professionalism, listening skills, skills in mental health and stability did not differentiate the two professionals. In general, while psychologists were found to be warmer and more caring than psychiatrists, they were still viewed as being less capable in dealing with the more serious disorders. However, with more psychologists working in mental institutions, only time will tell if such a stereotype will remain true.

Tessler, Gamache and Fisher (1991) interviewed patients who were discharged from state hospitals or 24-hour crisis care facilities in major cities of Ohio. They were asked to name family members who had been supportive during their mental illness. Four hundred nine family members were interviewed. All of the respondents were asked whether during the course of the patient's illness they had ever met or conversed with the patient's psychiatrist, psychologist, social worker, nurse, case manager, or other mental health professional on any matter pertaining to the patient's care. For each contact relatives were asked how satisfied they were with what was accomplished. Psychiatrists, who accounted for 27 percent of the 1,198 recent and past contacts, were identified most often in conjunction with contacts concerning medication (47% of all contacts were concerned with medication). Psychologists were most frequently contacted in conjunction with family therapy and the patients' behavioral problems. A one-way analysis of variance indicated that there were significant differences between the satisfaction on ratings for contact with various types of professionals. Respondents were satisfied with their contacts with psychologists, followed by nurses, case managers, social workers and psychiatrists. Thus the most satisfaction and least alienation were associated with psychologists and the least satisfaction and most alienation were associated with psychiatrists. According to these authors, past studies have shown that the strongest factor influencing family satisfaction was the occurrence of emotionally supportive interaction. This may explain why the highest percentage of respondents were very satisfied with family therapy. Again the use of psychotropic drugs by psychiatrists did not seem to make them popular with the families. It should be noted that this study was carried on by the Department of Sociology of the University of Massachusetts, Amherst and published in *Hospital and Community Psychiatry*, a psychiatric journal.

The July 1993 issue of the *American Psychologist* has a timely article (Murstein and Fontaine) on the public's knowledge about psychologists and other mental health professionals. This study incorporated three attributes: (1) the use of a random sample rather than the sample of convenience usually used in previous studies, (2) A larger number of mental health workers besides psychiatrists, (3) an examination of the public's experience with a mental health professional. Unfortunately out of 700 questionnaires which were mailed to New London County, Ct. residents, only 14.8% could be used. A large number of letters (92) were returned as undeliverable. The following are some of the findings. Compared to the other mental health professionals, specific knowledge about psychologists was rather poor. This is certainly understandable, since there are almost 50 different divisions of the American Psychological Association with their own specialties. Physicians and clergymen topped the list regarding their functions. In spite of the doubts shown about the function of the psychologist, as compared to the psychiatrist more respondents (24) indicated that they would consult a psychologist for mental health reasons, while the number for the psychiatrist would be 20. The type of mental health professionals most frequently recommended to a friend would be the marriage and family counselor, with psychologists, psychiatrists, physicians, members of the clergy, psychotherapists and social workers following in that order. Here again we see that the psychologist is preferred to the psychiatrist for personal problems as well as for referrals for friends. Respondents were asked how comfortable they would feel contacting each of the nine types of mental health professionals. The top of the list included the physician, the psychologist and the clergyperson, and the bottom of the list included the psychiatrist, the psychiatric nurse and the telephone counselor. Thus respondents did feel significantly more comfortable seeing a psychologist than a psychiatrist. Those who have seen mental health professionals in the past are more likely to recommend a psychologist than are those who have not seen one. According to Murstein and Fontaine (1993) the greater comfortableness of the respondents with psychologists compared to other trained mental health professionals suggests an increasing role for the former. These authors remarked that psychiatrists are unlikely to fade away, since they are the only ones who dispense drugs, but their role as "talking" psychotherapists is diminishing while their role as pill prescribers is increasing. It would appear from our review that this latter role does not make patients comfortable with psychiatrists. As we have seen, psychiatrists finished far down the list in comfortableness. One of the possible explanations given by Murstein and Fontaine is that psychiatrists have been trained in the authority-doctor-passive-patient model, whereas most psychologists work in a more egalitarian way with their clients. The authors however further indicated that as psychologists continue to make in-roads into what was once a totally medical/psychiatric jurisdiction (e.g., hospital privileges, the commitment of patients to hospitals, and drug prescriptions), the uncomfortableness favoring psychologists over psychiatrists may be erased. In conclusion, Murstein and Fontaine (1993) believe that there is a rising popularity of psychologists at the expense of psychiatrists. In view of the small number of respondents they suggest that the next round of research will render a verdict on the accuracy of their speculation. This research was financed in part by a grant from the Connecticut College psychology department.

In the original version of this paper, I expressed the hope that the American Psychological Association, with its tremendous financial resources, could confirm the verdict that psychology is a "talking" profession by conducting a large scale study and at the same time confirm the fact that the general consumer in general is less likely to accept psychotropic drugs by psychiatrists for his mental problems. This becomes all the more important in view of the efforts of a number of influential psychologists who are trying through legislative action to get prescription privileges for psychologists.

It seems that such a study was conducted by the American Psychological Association but it was not given the publicity that such a study deserved. I was able to get a copy by serendipity. The title of the research is, "Survey of general population of the USA on prescription privileges for psychologists." This survey was carried out by Frederick/Schneiders, a market research organization. The study consisted of telephone calls to 1,000 adults nationwide. The interviews were conducted between November 20 and November 23, 1992. Let me summarize the findings. The main question was whether Americans support "allowing psychologists to prescribe medication for their patients after completing additional training" (p. 2). College graduates (53%) support prescription privileges for psychologists, 39% oppose it and 8% don't know. The figures for high school graduates are 62, 31 and 7 percent respectively. However, what is more significant is the rest of the survey regarding medication and the feelings about the causes of mental disorders. In the APA survey, again for the college-educated respondent, 68% believe that the most important action to take in overcoming a mental health problem is "helping the person understand the personal and social situations that led to the problem," 10% would like "to foster responsibility," and only 12% believe that medication would be required. The least effective argument with consumers, in support of prescription privileges for psychologists is the fact that "nurses and other groups with less training in mental health than psychologists are safely prescribing medication." Fifty-three percent felt that this is not a good argument, 25% felt that it was somewhat good, and 15% felt it was a very good argument. It should be noted that this is one of the strongest arguments used by pro-drugs psychologists, that is, that other non-medical professions are able to prescribe.

Another interesting finding is that one-in-six Americans (16%) think that "most serious mental health problems are the result of a physical problem such as chemical imbalance" (p. 5). In view of the large scale efforts on the part of the psychiatric establishment, through their publications and the popular news media who reports on them, to persuade the public of the organicity of almost every type of mental disorder, I am delighted to see that the general public cannot easily be duped into this ideology.

The face sheet of the report indicates the following, "This report was received by the APA Board of Directors in December, 1992, with no further action. It does not represent an official policy position of the APA." I wonder about the significance of the last sentence.

CONCLUSIONS

While all of the studies reviewed are not comparable because of sampling differences, the type of questions asked, and the methodology used, there seems to be a consistent finding that psychologists rate very well with the general public and with other mental health professionals, while psychiatrists seem to have an image problem. While the number of psychologists is increasing, there seems to be a recruiting problem in psychiatry with many residencies left unfilled. What was most revealing in two large-scale studies by Cormark Communication, Inc. in Canada and the Keckley group in Atlanta, both financed by psychiatry, is that the respondents in both surveys prefer to see a psychologist over a psychiatrist. In the Canadian study one reason for the reluctance to see a psychiatrist was they "are too ready to prescribe drugs." In one study it was found that contacts between relatives of patients with psychiatrists had been least satisfactory, and a large percentage of these contacts had to do with the medication of these patients. Is it possible that the general public is becoming more familiar with the limitations of what were considered once "miracle drugs" and more attuned to "talk therapies"? This was confirmed by the survey commissioned by the American Psychological Association when 1000 adult individuals were interviewed nationwide. It was found that the best treatment for psychological problems is to have an opportunity to talk about the personal and social situations that led to these problems. Only 12% believed that drugs are the treatment of choice.

The studies reviewed in this paper should, for all intents and purposes, enhance the self-evaluation of psychologists; therefore, they should not consider their profession as inferior to psychiatry. The latter profession seems to be suffering in its popularity among the general public and in potential candidates for the profession. However, there are recent efforts on the part of the profession of psychiatry (Sanua, 1989) to deemphasize the medical model with drugs being the primary treatment modality. An article written in *Psychiatric News* (7/3/92) carries the following title, "Don't replace psychotherapy with a pill, experts remind public-sector psychiatrists" (p. 13). The article includes the following statement by Harold I. Eist: "I can't tell you how many times I've heard from inner-city patients 'Doc, don't give me a pill; I need someone to talk to.'" In the same article John C. Nemiah, editor of the *American Journal of Psychiatry,* raises the question as to "how psychiatrists are going to maintain sensitivity to the individual needs of the patients, when there is so much pressure to achieve the fast-acting, fairly quantifiable results so often provided by medication?" (p. 13).

Regarding the studies of the public image of psychologists, there seems to be a hodge-podge of small studies supported by limited grants from small departments of psychology. The psychiatric establishment has been willing to use some of their resources to get a better picture of the public's perception of psychiatry, while psychologists except for the APA telephone survey, have not pursued the same efforts with regard to their own profession. In view of the persistent conflicts and confrontation with psychiatry which has been trying to demean the contribution of psychology, it is surprising that a profession well-known for its strength in research has not seen fit to counteract these efforts through a better public relations and public information effort. For the past few years, the writer has been collecting pronouncements made at psychiatric conferences and conventions where pessimistic feelings have been expressed about psychiatry. Here are a few of them:

1. How effective is psychiatry? (Dietz, 1981).
2. Conceptual ambiguities and morality in modem psychiatry (Stone, 1980).
3. Psychiatry rides madly in all directions (Grinker, 1964).
4. The social discrediting of psychiatry (Dietz, 1977).
5. The death of psychiatry (Torrey, 1974).

Compared to psychiatry, psychology is becoming more and more vibrant and enlarging its scope of activities as illustrated by the establishment of new organizations, like the American Psychology Society and the American Association of Applied and Preventive Psychology.

Psychologists do not need to add to their treatment armamentarium psychotropic drugs which are of doubtful benefit to enhance their status. As revealed by the reviewed studies, psychology should limit itself to its humanistic and interpersonal approach to deal with people's problems. Psychology has come a long way from its laboratory roots to a respectable profession of helping people with their psychological skills. We can do better than psychiatrists. Let us not sell our professional birthright for a mess of pharmaceutical pottage.

REFERENCES

Alperin, R. M. & A. Benedict, (1985). College students: perceptions of psychiatrists, psychologists, and social workers–a comparison. *Psychological Reports,* 57, 547-548.

Buie, J. (1988). Brief attacks decision in California hospital issue. *The A.P.A. Monitor,* 19, (12), 22.

Canadian survey uncovers public's perceptions about psychiatry: stigma is hard to kill. *Psychiatric News,* XXIV, (10), 1989.

Cody, P. (1993). Residents matching in psychiatry continued to decline. *Psychiatric News,* XXVII (7), 1-20.

DeLeon, P. H., Folen, R. A., Jennings, F. L. Willis, D. J. & Wright, R. H. (1991). The case for prescription privileges: A logical evolution of professional practice. *Journal of Clinical Psychology,* 20(3), 254-267.

Dietz, P. E. (1977). Social discrediting of psychiatry. *American Journal of Psychiatry,* 134, 1356-1360.

Dietz, J. (1981). How effective is psychiatry? *Boston Globe,* April 21, 1981, p. 48.

Don't replace psychotherapy with a pill experts remind public-sector psychiatrists? *Psychiatric News,* XXVII, (3), July, 1992.

Dörken, H. (1990). Malpractice claim experience of psychologists: Policy issues, cost comparisons with psychiatrists, and prescription privilege implications. *Professional Psychology: Research and Practice,* 21, (2), 50-52.

Farley, F. (1993). The second century inaugural convention. *The A.P.A Monitor,* 24, (7), 3.

Grinker, R. R. Sr. (1964). Psychiatry rides madly in all directions. *Archives of General Psychiatry,* 10, 228-237.

Janik, A. & Kubickova, N. (1990). Stereotyp pri hodnoceni prestize lekarskych oboru. Stereotyping in evaluating the prestige of medical specialties. *Cesk-Psychiatrie,* 86, 73-79.

Kingsbury, S. J. (1987). Cognitive difference between clinical psychologists and psychiatrists. *American Psychologists,* 42, 152-156.

Koeske, G. F., Koeske, R. D. & Malinger, J. (1993). Perception of professional competence: cross disciplinary ratings of psychologist, social worker and psychiatrist. *American Journal of Orthopsychiatry,* 63, 45-54.

Murstein, B. I. & Fontaine, P. A. (1993). The public's knowledge about psychologists and other mental health professionals. *American Psychologist,* 48, (7), 839-845.

Neimeyer, G. J. & Walling, C. C. (1990). Perceived social influence in mental health, the professionals' perspective. *Social Behavior & Personality,* 18, 217-224.

Orne, M. T. (1980). Should psychiatrists be medically trained? Let's consider the alternatives in light of what the psychiatrist does. In J. P. Brady & H. K. H. Brodie (Eds.), *Psychiatry at the crossroads.* Philadelphia: The Saunders Press.

Psychiatry: Fact and perceptions. (1991, January) *National Register,* 16, (4), p. 19.

Rosario Webb, A. & Ramsay Speer, J. (1986). Prototype of a profession: psychology's public image. *Professional Psychology: Research and Practice* 17, (1), 5-9.

Rosario Webb, A. (1989). What's in a question? Three methods for investigating psychology's public image. *Professional Psychology: Research and Practice,* 20, (5), 301-304.

Sanua, V. (1989). Reflections on the status of psychiatry by psychiatrists. Midwinter Conference of Div. 29, 42, 43 of A.P.A. San Antonio Texas, Feb. 23rd, 1991.

Sanua, V. (1990). A history of "miracle" cures in the treatment of mental disorders. I. The age of shock therapies, II. The age of psychotropic drugs. Presented at the European Congress of Psychology, Budapest, Hungary, July 1990.

Sanua, V. (1993). A psychologist critically evaluates the profession of psychiatry in the U.S.A. In L. Communian and U. P. Gielen (Eds.), *Advancing psychology and its application: International Perspectives.* Milan: Franco Angeli Publishers.

Sanua, V. (1993a). Psychotropic drugs: Prescription for disasters, a review of the literature on the side-effects of psychiatric drugs. in press *Psychological Reports.*

Schindler, F., Berren, M. R., Hannah, M. T., Beigel, A. & Santiago, J. M. (1987).

How the public perceives psychiatrists, psychologists, nonpsychiatric physicians, and members of the clergy. *Professional Psychology: Research and Practice,* 18, (4), 371-376.

Stone, A. A. (1980). Presidential address: Conceptual ambiguities and morality in modern psychiatry. *American Journal of Psychiatry,* 137, 887-891.

Survey of general population of the United States on prescription privileges for psychologists. (November 1992). Prepared for the American Psychological Association by Frederick/Schneiders, Washington, D.C.

Tessler, R. C., Gamache, G. M. & Fisher G. A. (1991). Pattern of contact of patients' families with mental health professionals and attitude towards professionals. *Hospital Community Psychiatry,* 42, 429-35.

Torrey, E. F. (1974). *The death of psychiatry.* New York, NY: Penguin Books.

Warner, R. (1979). Racial and sexual bias in psychiatric diagnosis. *The Journal of Nervous and Mental Diseases,* 167, 303-310.

Webb, W. L. & Edwards, M. B., (1982). Psychiatry and medicine: marriage or divorce? In R. C. W. Hall (Ed.), *Psychiatry in crisis.* (73-84). New York: Sp. Medical and Scientific Books.

Wood, W., Jones, M. & Benjamin, L. T. Jr., (1986). Surveying psychology's public image. *American Psychologists,* 41, (9), 947-953.

Wright, R. & Spielberger, C. D. (1989). Psychiatry declares war on psychology. Letter to A.P.A. membership.

Psychotherapy with "Schizophrenia": Analysis of Metaphor to Reveal Trauma and Conflict

Richard Shulman

SUMMARY. Use of a medical or disease model of "schizophrenia" or "psychosis" often blinds us to seeing the metaphorical or poetic use of language in these conditions. Exploration of those metaphorical and camouflaged communications often uncovers poignant and relevant conflicts and traumas. After reviewing critiques of biological attempts at explanation, therapy case examples are given to exemplify a narrative approach to understanding functional "psychosis." *[Article copies available from The Haworth Document Delivery Service: 1-800-342-9678.]*

Actually, often the only thing "wrong" (as it were) with the so-called schizophrenic is that he speaks in metaphors unacceptable to his audience, in particular to his psychiatrist. . . . When persons imprisoned in mental hospitals speak of "rape" and "murder," they use inappropriate figures of speech which signify that they suffer from thought disorders; when psychiatrists call their prisons "hospitals," their prisoners "patients," and their "patients'" desire for lib-

Richard Shulman, PhD, was educated at Wesleyan University, the University of Michigan and the University of Toledo. He practices in Hartford, Connecticut, where he has done individual, family and group therapy for ten years with people given a variety of "psychotic" and "schizophrenic" diagnoses. He has presented papers on this subject at numerous conferences including the National Convention of the American Psychological Association.

[Haworth co-indexing entry note]: "Psychotherapy with 'Schizophrenia': Analysis of Metaphor to Reveal Trauma and Conflict." Shulman, Richard. Co-published simultaneously in *The Psychotherapy Patient* (The Haworth Press, Inc.) Vol. 9, No. 3/4, 1996, pp. 75-106; and: *Psychosocial Approaches to Deeply Disturbed Persons* (eds: Peter R. Breggin, and E. Mark Stern) The Haworth Press, Inc., 1996, pp. 75-106. Single or multiple copies of this article are available from The Haworth Document Delivery Service [1-800-342-9678, 9:00 a.m. - 5:00 p.m. (EST)].

77

erty "disease," the psychiatrists are not using figures of speech, but are stating facts.

Thomas Szasz (1976, p. 14)

Meanings alter in the service of emotional needs; and when a person's acceptability to himself and others is threatened, when no way out of an irreconcilable dilemma can be found, and when all paths into the future seem blocked, there is still a way. One can simply alter his perceptions of his own needs and motivations and those of others; one can abandon causal logic or change the meanings of events; one can regress . . . In short, one can become schizophrenic.

Communication is of the essence, and the patient is weaned from his autistic preoccupations and his idiosyncratic communications by the therapist's ability to hear and understand what the patient wishes to say even while he seeks to conceal through the use of idiosyncratic metaphor and cryptic associations.

Theodore Lidz (1973, p. 10 & p. 103)

/some would have us/ . . . turn relatively quickly to the latest information from such scientific fields as behavior genetics, biochemistry, psychopharmacology, epidemiology, and so on to find reassuring evidence that the schizophrenic patient is, after all, qualitatively different from truly human beings; so that it is pointless to risk one's own sanity by persisting in this disturbingly conflict-ridden effort to work psychoanalytically with him.

Harold Searles (1975b, p. 226)

. . . even the most "crazy," manifestations of schizophrenia come to reveal meaningfulness and reality-relatedness not only as transference-reactions to the therapist, but, even beyond this, as delusional identifications with real aspects of the therapist's own personality . . .

Harold Searles (1965, p. 34)

One can repeat specifically with respect to the psychoanalytic therapy of schizophrenia, as well as other psychosocial treatments,

Freud's comments about psychoanalysis, that, in Mark Twain's words, "The reports of my death are greatly exaggerated."

Bertram Karon (1989, pp. 146-7)

Let's imagine that we have just begun seeing a young man in therapy after he has ended a program with another therapist. He comes late to an initial session, mentioning that he was delayed trying to visit his old therapist, but she wasn't there. If he next mentioned that he'd heard a news story about a woman who abandoned her baby in a dumpster, stating that he thought she should be shot, we might begin to hypothesize that the vignette about the baby held some relevance to his feelings about his current situation. This hypothesis might be strengthened if his other comments seemed to coalesce around similar themes, such as telling you how silent you've been, or criticizing inhospitable aspects of your office.

In this regard we might be informed by the writings of Harold Searles, Robert Langs and others who view a patient's verbalizations as frequently being thematically relevant to the therapeutic context, or as being unconscious supervision. These and other writers alert us to attend to the metaphorical and thematic relevance of the patient's associations—with particular reference to the current state of the therapeutic relationship—and therefore to put less emphasis on the manifest content of what is said. Given this perspective, we would not be put off from our therapeutic task if the client used metaphors that we judged to be unrealistic on a manifest or surface level. For example, they might state that they *were* a baby in a dumpster, or tell us that they were an aborted fetus. Or perhaps they might tell us that they were a crew member on the spaceship "Juan Doe." Only later we might learn that "Juan Doe" was the name of the infamous "garbage barge" that was denied entry to numerous ports. If we made this simple transition to listening thematically and metaphorically, and to listening without undue emphasis as to whether what was said sounded "unrealistic," "psychotic" or initially incomprehensible, we would be doing what we have been told we can't or shouldn't do—therapeutic exploration with people whom we typically call "schizophrenic."[1]

FOCUS OF THIS PAPER

This paper aims to resurrect debate about several questions related to the conditions commonly known as "schizophrenia" or "psychosis," and to point to clinical and research evidence which suggest that our current predominant models for understanding these conditions may be blinding us to other, more cogent, perspectives for understanding them. Specifically, our reliance on the imagery of "mental" or physical illness and disease has contributed to discounting a more linguistic, narrative or metaphorical analysis of the communications that we label as "psychotic symptoms."

My own conviction in this regard is directly linked to my experience as a psychotherapist. With great regularity I have found it increasingly possible, throughout the course of discussion (therapy) with a "psychotic" person, to understand certain symbolization used in their talk, and to see how such poetic or camouflaged language may relate quite compellingly to previously unexplored personal dilemmas or conflicts, or to previously undisclosed trauma. With regularity I have seen that once reasonable attention and discussion is devoted to those metaphorical uses of language (what might be called the "symptoms": the "thought disorders," "delusions" or "hallucinations") and to their referents (the traumas and conflicts), that the "symptoms" fade from prominence, and are replaced by a more direct discussion of the problematic traumas and conflicts themselves.

But though these therapy experiences form the basis for this paper, I will first present some more general criticisms of the "mental health" professions' prevailing and predominant approach to the problem of "psychosis," in order to show just how tenuous and unsupported those more biological attempts at explanation are. Some organizations urge us to define some behaviors as "symptoms" of "mental illness" or of a probable but as yet unproven brain disease. We are exhorted to "learn to see the sickness" (as in one prominent advertising campaign). But I propose that this is akin to being urged to learn to see the emperor's new clothes. That is, we are being urged to blind ourselves to the "nakedness" (the lack of substantiation of the medical metaphors and hypotheses), just as we are being urged to ignore how some people (the "psychotic patients") are trying to communicate (albeit ambivalently and in a camouflaged manner) with us.

We must remember that people receive the diagnosis of "schizophrenic" or "psychotic" on the basis of their words or behavior, not based on the status of their brains. It is, of course, not impossible that future medical research will show us some substantive substrate of explanatory biological fabric for "psychosis." However, we should not lose sight of the fact that we are being exhorted to see what is not yet established (that these are at root medical "diseases"). We are being tacitly asked to collude in ignoring certain alternative and, I believe, cogent explanations ("naked facts") which we also *could* see in front of our eyes.

In the Hans Christian Andersen tale, the strategy used by the tailors to gain compliance with their shared falsehood was to let it be known that those who could not see the fine clothes they were producing for the Emperor were either fools or unfit for their posts. Similarly, we can see parallels in the subtle coercion of the "mental health" professions. We are exhorted and pressured to see the "sickness," the "mental illness," and to use language suggesting disease, disability, mental incompetence, insanity and biological illness. We are inherently asked to blind ourselves to the possibility that there is camouflaged communication in what the people we call "psychotic" are saying to us; and to the possibility that there may be meaning in their "madness."

QUESTIONING "SCHIZOPHRENIA" AS A DISEASE

The conception of "schizophrenia" as disease is questionable from several perspectives, some simply by analogy or comparison. Elsewhere in work with troubled people, we accept that people can say things which we don't comprehend at first, can make statements which seem manifestly at odds with reality, can deny certain accepted assumptions about their identity, their experience or their memory. They can do these things in a way which seems bizarre or initially inexplicable to a "rational" or relatively "objective" observer. Yet we need not resort to exclusively or predominantly medical hypotheses to explain such discrepancies. For example, in the condition typically termed "multiple personality disorder," a person may tell us that they are five years old and named Sue, or five minutes later, that they are 30 years old and named Sylvia. They may state that these two entities have distinctly different memories and experiences and no knowledge of each other. Since these descriptions are at odds with what we call consensual reality, they could be labeled "psychotic."

The literature on this form of human functioning and experience (or "psychopathology") points with near unanimity to potentially formative childhood experiences which help account for these "psychotic" descriptions. Such childhood experiences are commonly known and documented by now. Typically they involve repeated and cruel infliction of torture, sexual and physical abuse, or exposure to a traumatic event such as the witnessing of the violent death of a loved one (Putnam et al., 1986). These powerful personal experiences, many of which are secret or unrevealed at the outset of therapy, help us to understand how "psychotic" characterological configurations could be comprehended as adaptations to overwhelming stress. They are "psychotic" configurations in the sense that people describe their identity and experience in ways which are manifestly at odds with consensual reality. As Rosenberg (1984) has pointed out, we call actions, behavior or people "psychotic" when we initially can't comprehend their logic or point of view, and when we conclude that they are inherently incomprehensible.

There has been some evidence of physiological correlates of aspects of multiple personality disorder (Braun, 1983), and I am not arguing that researchers should not investigate any human problem from any perspective (sociological, chemical, anatomical, religious, economic, etc.) which could conceivably prove illuminating or helpful. But certainly the case of "multiple personality disorder" alerts us to the potentially central importance of linguistic, psychotherapeutic, narrative or experiential studies of people whom at first we might label "psychotic" (since we have not yet made sense of their words and behavior). Along these lines, Sarbin (1986) points to the dangers of tacitly accepting a mechanistic or positivistic approach to science, which may then preclude productive contextualist or narrative explorations that can contribute to our understanding of psychological phenomena.

Given what we know of "multiple personality disorder," we might then posit that people adapt to stress in different ways. Some people get headaches, some get anxious, some become sad and forlorn, some take their frustrations out on others, and some people talk or describe themselves in ways that at first seem incomprehensible to others, or report having experiences that seem inexplicable or unrealistic ("psychotic"). Certainly reports of "hallucinations" by hostages who have been isolated while their lives were threatened seem to support these inferences (Siegel, 1984).

Those who promulgate the metaphor of "mental illness" usually ignore or deemphasize "diagnostic" categories which link clear experiential precipitants with the "illnesses." We are less likely to hear "multiple personality disorder" or "post-traumatic stress disorder" described as diseases or "mental illnesses." Instead, the term "mental illness" tends to be applied to situations in which peoples' behavior or statements about themselves initially appear to be perplexing or unexplained in terms of their life experience. Such medical language often implies that there is some unspecified biological disorder, or perhaps some biological marker which is yet to be discovered, which would account for the unusual, disturbing or incomprehensible thoughts or behavior.

In fact, Thomas Szasz's (1976) critique of the conceptualization of "schizophrenia" as a "disease" emphasizes this frequently and conveniently forgotten link in reasoning about "mental illness": the typical medical model of disease elucidation involves confirmation of the histo-pathology (tissue pathology) or malfunction that underlies some humanly unwanted or deleterious symptom or complaint. He notes that in the case of "schizophrenia," no underlying tissue pathology has ever been demonstrated. Instead, the "discovery" of the disease rather was its "invention," when attention was called to a cluster of behaviors which seemed to frequently coexist.

Elsewhere, Szasz (1987) incorporates the evidence compiled by the "experts on diseases of the body, . . . pathologists." He cites pathology textbooks to show that although "ever since the earliest days of psychiatry, psychiatrists have *claimed* that mental diseases are brain diseases; *that pathologists have never been able to confirm these claims*" (p. 71, emphasis in original). He concludes that "psychiatrists ought to convince pathologists that schizophrenia is a brain disease before they take it upon themselves to tell the public that it is such a disease or try to silence those who disagree with them on this crucial issue" (p. 73).

The central point here, which we frequently keep ourselves blind to, is that no one has ever been diagnosed as "psychotic" or "schizophrenic" on the basis of anything other than a judgment of their words and behavior. Neither a CAT scan, an autopsy nor a test of neurotransmitters has ever been used to diagnose this "disease," nor could they be, because there is no such demonstrated or reliable biological substrate. Burrell (1992) has pointed to the specification of the DSM-III-R, noting that "schizophrenia" can only be diagnosed when . . . "It cannot be established that an organic factor initiated and maintained the disturbance" (p. 192). Alternatively, "when a person presents with symptoms characteristic of Schizophrenia, the diagnosis can be made only when the clinician concludes, after an appropriate evaluation, that no organic factor (such as a psychoactive substance or a brain tumor) can be established to have initiated and maintained the disturbance" (p. 22). (See also Szasz (1987) on this issue.)

What Szasz articulates as a logical critique of our blind acceptance of the term "schizophrenia" as a disease, Sarbin and Mancuso (1980) reinforce through their critical review of much of the prominent recent literature which purports to support the viability of "schizophrenia" as a useful and distinct psychological term, and the literature that is usually cited to substantiate the view that "schizophrenia" is a medical diagnosis with a biological substrate. Like Szasz, they emphasize that repeated attempts to scientifically shore up the diagnostically distinct psychological concept of "schizophrenia," or to find definitive or replicable biological markers of any tissue pathology, have consistently failed. Among other powerful critiques, they point out the regularity with which researchers who claimed to have identified a psychological or biological correlate of "schizophre-nia" were generalizing from published findings of small but statistically significant differences between the arithmetic means for *groups* of "schizo-phrenic" and "normal" samples. There were often substantial overlaps in the data for each group, and often great variability in the data within the "schizophrenic" samples. The authors point to the fallacy of assuming that such findings, which were not routinely replicated, supported the notion that the groups could be definitively differentiated by use of the variables being studied. Many of these studies violated fundamental tenets of research by failing to control for disguised aspects of the experimental context, such as the use of major tranquilizers, or they failed to control for other potentially intervening variables, such as intelligence, level of education, the effects of institutionalization or patienthood experiences. I will not summarize their work here, but I urge that their critique *(Schizo-phrenia: Medical diagnosis or moral verdict?)* be read by those who tacitly accept the disease model of "schizophrenia" as being either log-ically appropriate or confirmed by research. Sarbin later summarizes and extends these arguments (1990, 1992).

Similarly, Bentall, Jackson and Pilgrim (1988) review prominent psy-chiatric research and conclude that there is strong reason to consider other approaches to studying the amorphous and indiscrete phenomena we call "schizophrenic." Their review convinces them that, "Not only is it impossible to decide whether schizophrenia is a disease or a form of social deviance without first identifying such an entity, but no meaningful research can be carried out comparing schizophrenics to others without first establishing the reliability and validity of the schizophrenia diagno-sis" (p. 305). After reviewing the inconsistent neurological, biochemical and psychological research, they emphasize the lack of usefulness of "schizophrenia" as a scientific category. They remind us that the "history of science is littered with examples in which progress has been impeded by the continued use of invalid categories leading to the persistent asking of the wrong questions" (p. 317). The authors point to economic, political and primarily guild interests (mostly involving organized psychiatry and psychology) which may perpetuate such invalid diagnoses. These same interests may promote a relatively blind "article of faith" in the potential for future, more refined research to *eventually* document the validity of "schizophrenia" as a label or as a medical/biological diagnosis or entity. Their review argues for "abandoning the 'schizophrenia' concept" in favor of research into more discretely identified "psychotic symptoms." Persons' (1986) paper, "The advantages of studying psychological phenomena rather than psychiatric diagnoses" makes similar and complementary arguments.

Boyle (1990) goes into great detail to review flaws in logic and research design in many studies which profess to strengthen the concept of "schizophrenia" as a valid psychological or diagnostic category, or especially to portray it as a disease. In one chapter of her book *Schizophrenia: A scientific delusion?*, she critically reviews the claims of evidence for a "genetic" factor in schizophrenia based on adoption and twin studies, revealing the paucity of research support for the predominant biological claims. She, like many authors cited here, also questions "Why has /the concept of/ 'schizophrenia' survived?" Similar critiques of the research claiming to establish the biological basis of "schizophrenia" are available (Breggin, 1991; Cohen, 1989; Cohen & Cohen, 1986; Karon, 1991; Karon, 1992; Lidz, 1973; Lidz & Blatt, 1983; Rose, 1984; Sass, 1992).

Breggin's (1983) critical review of a segment of the literature on major tranquilizers undermines a corollary to the medical model of schizophrenia. He points out the historical falsification of the effects of major tranquilizers that led to their inaccurate labeling as "anti-psychotic" drugs. By reviewing key research and recounting the historical derivation of these drugs, he shows how their primary effect is tranquilizing, sedating, or in his estimation "brain-disabling." He demonstrates that, far from being a specific treatment for a supposedly identifiable neurochemical malfunction or disease, these drugs are cognitively repressive and disorienting agents that affect all people ("normal" or not) as well as animals. He points out how other medical specialties recognize this; only within psychiatry are these drugs relabeled and promoted with claims that they are a specific treatment for a specific illness. For example, in emergency medicine, major tranquilizers are recognized as a sedating agent for any uncontrolled, disruptive or belligerent patient (Clinton et al., 1987).

Breggin's (1991) *Toxic Psychiatry* also summarizes and critiques aspects of the literature which purport to identify "schizophrenia" as a disease, or to portray major tranquilizers as specific remedies for that disease. He supports the reasoning of Sarbin and Mancuso (1980) by pointing to evidence that the abnormalities that sometimes have been shown to statistically differentiate groups of "schizophrenics" from normals on brain scans, or with regard to neurotransmitters, are probably not innate anatomical or chemical markers of "schizophrenia." Instead, he argues that at least some of those abnormalities are evidence of the iatrogenically-induced damaging effects of major tranquilizers, particularly associated with long term consumption.

Rappaport et al. (1978a), in examining research evidence of "schizophrenics for whom drugs may be unnecessary or contraindicated" (p. 100), summarize findings of phenothiazine effects "such as decreased sensory and psychological sensitivity, decreased problem-solving ability and a decreased ability to learn" (p. 107). In another review of evidence questioning whether these drugs are more than "palliative," Rappaport (1978b) reviews "instances in which the use of antischizophrenic medication has little or no effect and where its use is probably unnecessary" (p. 223). He states that "the numbers of individuals involved cannot be considered by any stretch of the imagination to be insignificant" (p. 223). Though he later concludes "that antischizophrenia drugs are extremely valuable in favorably modifying unwanted psychological symptoms in some patients" (p. 229), his review also reconfirms "patient complaints about being 'held down' or being in a chemical straitjacket" (p. 223). Cohen and Cohen (1986) acknowledge that many "patients" take such drugs willingly because "they feel that the calming effects are worth a degree of discomfort or diminished alertness" (p. 23). However, they underscore Coleman's (1984) crucial distinction: "it makes a difference whether a patient takes drugs because he or she finds them helpful or because the patient believes that modern science has discovered a brain abnormality that can be treated with drugs" (Cohen & Cohen, 1986, p. 23).

I have witnessed psychiatrists warning colleagues to not openly use terms such as "chemical restraints" or "major tranquilizers" in describing such drugs, for fear that certain psychiatric practices might be criticized. So, we are marshalled to deny what we see. But who among us in our professional work has not seen these drugs used for just that purpose—to subdue or sedate unwanted, unruly or initially incomprehensible behavior? Why is it that in some areas of psychiatric practice we are pressured to describe these drugs in a biased manner? Again we can see the relevance of the "Emperor's New Clothes" metaphor. Those who disagree with the conventional view of "anti-psychotic" medication are seen as "fools" or "unfit for their posts."

Breggin (1991) also provides a lengthy historical and investigative description of the guild competition among mental health professions, and particularly of the increasing corporate alliance between the profession of psychiatry and the pharmaceutical industry. Those two groups in particular can have a mutual interest in describing human problems of confusing, disturbing or disruptive behavior as if they were primarily reducible to organic malfunctions. However, as we have seen, such organic substrates are neither consistently substantiated by research nor confirmed in the particular "patient." Yet, those theories do provide the rationale for the use of medication (which Breggin continues to demonstrate, provides a basically "brain disabling" effect), and a rationale for the position of psychiatry as the authoritative force in explaining and managing troubled or troubling people within society.

Along similar lines, Scull (1975) supplies an informative historical account of how, in the nineteenth century, "that segment of the medical profession which we now call psychiatry . . . acquired a monopolistic power to define and treat lunatics" (p. 218). He points out that there was at that time "a lack of any real knowledge base which would have given the medical profession a rationally defensible claim to possess expertise vis-à-vis insanity" (p. 222). Hence certain implicit parallels may be drawn historically and sociologically to the professional debates and guild interests of our own time. Since the period Scull describes, it has been "the psychiatrists /who/ possess the ultimate power to assign one person to the status of being mentally ill, and to refuse the designation to another" (p. 221).

Leifer (1990) and Breggin (1991) describe instances in which vocal critics of those biological theories and disease models have been threatened and censured, both by curtailment of teaching opportunities and terminations of employment in academia, and by attempts to strip professionals of their licenses. Colleagues inform me that biologically-oriented professionals experienced similar professional repression in the past, when psychosocial and psychoanalytic theories were more ascendant. Clearly, such squelching of debate and academic freedom is reprehensible in the service of anyone's views, and it is scandalous in terms of what information it provides and denies both to the public and to relevant clinicians.

SOME PSYCHOSOCIAL PERSPECTIVES ON "PSYCHOSIS"

Some writers have tried to make sense of "psychotic symptoms" from a more experiential perspective. Bettelheim (1956) worked with "psychotic" children and began to wonder about the sense of terror, the emotional and cognitive confusion, and the distortions of reality he perceived. He realized that he had seen such reactions previously in concentration camp inmates and survivors. He began to conceptualize these "symptoms" as "reactions to extreme situations," by which he meant traumatic and overwhelming situations from which the person could not withdraw or escape. Support for such observations comes from other clinical areas. For a considerable time we have had documentation of traumatic combat situations which provoked "psychotic symptoms" (e.g., Grinker & Spiegel, 1945). Dohrenwend and Egri (1981) provide evidence that "symptomatology of schizophrenia observed in combat situations is indistinguishable from the symptoms of schizophrenia observed in patients from civilian populations" (p. 17). They describe the stresses attendant to "prolonged exposure to heavy combat," reminding us that these "extreme situations" involve a loss of control in experiencing the "death of comrades, threat of one's own death or disablement . . . and being stripped of . . . social support" (p. 18).

Similarly, Siegel's (1984) inquiry into hostage situations which led to hallucinatory experiences, suggests that these experiences derive from "conditions of isolation, visual deprivation, restraint on physical movements, physical abuse, and threat of death" (p. 269). In attempting to understand which of the hostages had "hallucinations," he finds that "the critical combination appears to be the presence of both isolation *and* the threat of death" (p. 270).

Earlier in this paper, I pointed out the regularity with which people described as exemplifying multiple personality disorder later revealed excruciating instances or ongoing experiences of childhood trauma or abuse. In describing the evolution of his observations about life situations which contribute to "schizophrenia," Lidz (1973) states:

> Then, I noted during my residency that all of the schizophrenic patients under my care came from disturbed or very peculiar families. Indeed, sometimes after spending an hour or two with one or both of the patient's parents, I would wonder just how long my sanity or anyone's sanity would withstand living with these people, to say nothing of being raised by them. (p. 8)

> Interest in the family milieu in which schizophrenic patients grew up was stimulated further because close relatives of several patients, *who had not been taught that we were dealing with a disease of unknown etiology,* ignorantly explained to me just how the situation in the patient's family had driven the patient crazy. (p. 9, emphasis added)

Where Freud had conceptualized his patient's reports of incest as oedipal fantasies, Lidz's observations with these families led him to very different conclusions. Lidz's evidence suggested that "when not reflecting actual experiences, such reports occur when the patient's fantasy had been stimulated by a parent's near incestuous behavior or attitudes" (p. 112, note).

Karon (1991) expresses somewhat similar observations. He cites the research on "expressed emotion" (see for example Leff & Vaughn, 1980) and "parental communication deviance" in families of "schizophrenic patients" (research which is often associated supportively with Lidz's views), and continues:

In no case have I ever treated a schizophrenic whose life, as experienced, would not have driven me crazy. Where the therapeutically reconstructed material concerned externally observable events, it has been possible to confirm them. It is not isolated traumata, but continuing pressures, mediated through the resulting conscious and unconscious fantasy structures, which make human beings vulnerable. Whenever the family environment was unfortunate and the individual did not end up psychotic, there were always people outside the family who provided corrective identifications and experiences. Whenever the family environment was not unfortunate and the individual ended up psychotic, there were always traumatic experiences outside the family which were overwhelming. (Karon, 1991, p. 8)

He states his clinical experience that "in every case there are parent-child interactions, whose consequences are hurtful, but different overt behaviors occur in different families" (p. 7). But he also emphasizes that in previous theorizing and research, portrayals of "the schizophrenegenic mother were over-simplified and gross." Earlier (Karon & VandenBos, 1981) he had devoted considerable effort to contradicting the accusatory or guilt-ridden view that parents of "schizophrenics" were simply "criminal" or "evil." Lidz agrees:

The patient's illness is far more tragic to the parents than to the therapist, and their noxious influences upon the patient were not malevolent but rather the product of their own personal tragedies and their egocentric orientations. (p. 122)

Rosenberg (1984) examined the use of the term "insane" by experts and laymen, showing that both groups label a person's behavior or speech "insane" when they are unable to account for the protagonist's behavior from that person's perspective. However, Karon and VandenBos (1981) supply case examples of therapeutic exploration of "schizophrenics'" seemingly insane or incomprehensible verbalizations. They demonstrate that it is not an impossible task to begin to decipher some of the symbolism involved. For instance, they describe the case of a man who was frequently seemingly unprovokedly violent, who was often incoherent or silent, and who stated cryptically, "You swallow a snake, and then you stutter; you mustn't let anyone know about it" (p. 38). The authors show how verbal and symbolic investigation revealed that as a child this man had been regularly choked by a family member, had been incestuously raped, and later was orally/sexually involved with a priest. These experiences previously had been secret and undiscussed, and contributed to the man's subsequent speech impediment, as well as to his other formerly inscrutable behaviors and verbalizations.

The Karon and VandenBos book is recommended to any student of psychotherapy with "psychotic" patients, both for the illustrative symbolic case examples they discuss, and for their larger psychotherapy outcome research that documents the efficacy of psychotherapy in such situations. Additionally, they examine critical flaws in most of the previous psychotherapy research which had seemed to demonstrate the inefficacy of psychotherapy with "schizophrenics." Previous research frequently ignored the inexperience of the therapists and supervisors studied, often utilizing residents or therapists who had little experience with such "patients." Previous studies also used therapists who were involuntarily recruited to do psychotherapy with psychotic patients. Other flaws cited were the absence of either blind evaluation, or of long term follow-up measurement in the studies. Karon (1989) later updates and expands his critical review of studies which have compared the effects of psychotherapy with those of medication in working with "schizophrenics."

However, much as I urge critical reading of these cited works, it was not reading them that convinced me of the efficacy and importance of psychotherapeutic exploration of "psychotic" verbalizations or other "symptoms." Instead, I was first convinced through experiences in psychotherapy that were similar to those of Karon and VandenBos.

ILLUSTRATIVE THERAPY SESSIONS

First, let's consider some vignettes from a therapy session with a "nonpsychotic patient." (The following case examples are disguised for reasons of confidentiality). The man described at the beginning of this article had been in outpatient therapy with me for several months when he came to a session late. He said that he had stopped by his old therapist's office, but he had just missed her. Next he described a recent news story in which a woman had given birth to a child and had left the baby in a dumpster. He felt that she should be shot. He then mentioned that in his carpentry work he'd recently dealt with a customer who had moved into a house that was under construction and was not complete yet. He told me what a "dumb move" he thought that was. Then he pointed out that I wasn't saying much. I was reminded that more than once recently he had mentioned clocks or watches that "worked when they want to." I pointed out that he had mentioned not seeing his old therapist; that imagery had come up about a mother abandoning a child, and about someone going into a new situation that wasn't really prepared adequately, and that he'd referred to my quietness. I said that it made me wonder if there might be parallels between what he'd said and the situation of leaving his old therapy and starting with me. After being quiet for a while he shrugged as if to dismiss my comment, and then began to speak of a guy he'd paid to fix his car. He said that the guy had done a pretty good job, but then he'd jammed in a part, damaging the trunk. I thought it best to be quiet.

Many of us are exposed to this manner of listening in therapy. It is a conceptualization of the associations or verbalizations in therapy as being expressive (perhaps on an indirect or "unconscious" level) of the emotional reactions of the client, and perhaps with particular relevance to situations in the therapy. In this approach to psychodynamic understanding, most prominently discussed by both Searles and Langs, particular attention is given to seeing client communications as "derivative commentaries" (Langs, 1976) which express the client's emotional reactions to actual actions and attitudes of the therapist. From this perspective, the patient's associations are seen as unconscious supervision by which "the patient is therapist to his analyst" (Searles, 1975a). In the session just described, I believed that this man's associations may have held some relevance to his reaction to me and my seeming lack of involvement in the therapy. His subsequent vignette may also have expressed his reaction to, and partial criticism of, my comment. That is why I decided to be quiet. In later weeks, I noticed that this man spoke regularly of his tendency to jam on his brakes when driving on the highway, whenever he sensed he was being followed too closely.

In this approach to listening in psychotherapy, it is not of primary importance whether something a patient says is factually or realistically true or accurate. The job of the therapist is not conceptualized as being a judge of the ("manifest level") literal truth or accuracy of statements. Instead, statements are examined to try to appreciate levels of feeling and communication that may be more subtle, or harder to describe, more complicated, conflicted or ambivalent, perhaps less categorical, perhaps more dreamlike, more awesome, emotionally poignant, or unspeakable.

In the clinical situation just mentioned, the imagery of a car following too closely, or of something being jammed into someone's trunk, turned out to be a very apt symbolic or poetic expression of a central concern of this man. These images foreshadowed a gradual direct discussion of very real and formative traumatic sexual experiences he had had which contributed heavily to his difficulties with men in particular.

But once emphasis is given to listening to therapeutic communications from a metaphorical, symbolic perspective, any preoccupation with judging the literal accuracy of a person's statements becomes irrelevant. If a patient in a session chose to tell us that they *were* a baby in a dumpster, rather than simply relating a news item with a similar theme, should we abandon the search for the potential underlying meanings of such an assertion (since we judge the communication to be literally not true, and hence "psychotic")? Why would we understand the statement to be so radically different from what this man said to me?

By way of further comparison, in trying to understand a dream, we may scan the descriptions for potential personal or idiographic meanings, or their relevance to current situations. But most therapists wouldn't consider criticizing the seeming illogicalities of the dream imagery as a way of invalidating potential relevancies of the dream. Why would we therefore stop the search for metaphorical relevance in client communications generally, just because the communications may seem implausible, unrealistic, or "psychotic" on a manifest level?

Here is a brief example. A woman applied to return to therapy in the clinic where she had seen a male therapist years before. He had left the clinic and she had continued to work with him in a new setting. Part of the therapy had focused on her past history of sexual abuse. The therapist had encouraged her to confront her family about this secret. When she failed to follow some of the suggestions he felt were most important for her, he ended the therapy. She returned to the old clinic for an intake interview. To be helpful, the old therapist spoke with the intake worker, reviewing the course of the therapy and discussing the referral. In the intake interview, the patient spoke about her father. She said he ran a prostitution ring, and she also believed that he called ahead to any stores or other places where she went. She said that wherever she went, people had already been contacted by him.

In a subsequent staff meeting, the woman was given a psychotic diagnosis. The staff reasoned that there was no evidence in reality that her father ran a prostitution ring, and that her other concern, that anyone she met had already been contacted by him, seemed "paranoid." There were suggestions that she would only be appropriate for "treatment" by "medication" and not by "therapy."

Instead, the patient's cogent metaphorical communication describing pimping and procurement might have alerted staff to ways in which the actions of the previous therapist and of the intake worker may have been recreating traumatic patterns reminiscent of her sexual abuse. We might remember that the previous therapist *had* tried to run her life, at least to some extent, and he had eventually terminated her therapy when she wouldn't do what he said. Her reference to her father's intrusive communication similarly might have poignantly expressed her sense of violation or contamination at the communication between the old therapist and the intake worker.

Here is a condensed clinical example of how "psychotic" communications may be explored for their metaphorical relevance. I saw a young man in therapy who had recently been hospitalized on several occasions, in part for his disruptiveness and "hyper-religiosity." He had begun to stay up late at night, while living in his mother and step-sister's home, and he would preach to them from the Bible because he felt that he needed to get them to change. He thought perhaps he was Jesus Christ. At times he would be silent for long periods of time. He also said he sometimes had visions of people's faces being mangled or crushed. Only much later did he add that they were often the faces of his family.

Over the course of some family therapy sessions the man spoke of the devil being in his house, though some people might not know it, or might not want to talk about it. Certain sexual references were made as he described the devil coming into people's rooms at night. When such imagery had recurred, I questioned whether any devilish or sexual secrets had actually gone on in the home. Eventually, when this symbolism and my question had come up more than once, the step-sister asked if I meant something like the time she had put rubber bands and clamps on his genitals. She eventually revealed that she had secretly physically and sexually abused him for an ongoing period of time when they were left alone as children. She also related these acts to the beatings her mother secretly had given her. These revelations came out quite haltingly, over a long period of time, and were accompanied by expressions of her fear that she was responsible for driving her stepbrother crazy. She hinted repeatedly at her guilty feelings and looked to the patient for some confirmation or disagreement. He would avoid eye contact and become silent at such times. When pressed, he denied that she had hurt him, telling me privately that such abuse couldn't have happened because he didn't have a stepsister.

At one point the young man was required to have an appointment with a psychiatrist. He insisted to me that he did not want to be returned to prescriptions of major tranquilizers. I emphasized that he should feel free to tell the psychiatrist how he felt. When he had that meeting, it was noted in the chart that the man had said little and was seen as "catatonic," and that the psychiatrist next met with the man's mother and privately gave her medication for him.

At the next meeting with the family, the client began to speak of how he had cut up vitamin pills and had given them to a young relative to drink, unbeknownst to her, mixed with her juice. As he continued to talk, imagery of poison came up, and of coercion. His mother insisted that he was "talking crazy," and that no such events with juice and vitamins had happened. I suggested that perhaps his comments were relevant, pointing out the potential parallel with what had evidently happened with the psychiatrist, the mother and the medication. He then produced numerous stories of lurid, illegal and sometimes sexual activities that occurred around his home, that he knew of and that others either didn't know of or didn't want to speak of. Eventually the discussion led back again to the sexual abuse that had never been fully discussed. The mother discounted and disparaged her son's remarks, pointing out the manifest illogicalities in some of the stories he told. She hinted that she didn't want to continue such discussions, while simultaneously complaining that her son's feelings were "too bottled up" and that he didn't communicate enough. The stepsister, in the mother's absence, later revealed other previously secret incestuous contacts which had occurred in the family years ago, between other adults and herself and other children.

Here is another clinical example. I worked with a young woman who felt confused and vague about what her problems were, and why she had made several suicide attempts. She had been hospitalized numerous times and was viewed as "psychotic" each time. For months at a time she told me that it seemed inexplicable that she kept repeatedly and inescapably thinking of a guy in a leather jacket. She insisted that those thoughts were her only problem. However, she often had been hospitalized when she was very upset and felt certain that others were trying to kill her. She had told me that she had started years of intermittent hospitalizations following her father's abrupt death when she was a teenager. When her mother joined her for family therapy sessions, certain missing pieces were described.

The mother began to point out that, while she insisted that she had never minded her husband's actions, for years he had chosen to spend the vast majority of his free time with his daughter. He would bathe her and tuck her into bed at night, often falling asleep there in her bed. The mother then pointed out that his bathing of the girl had continued into her teenage years, and that the girl (client) should not have permitted this. It became increasingly clear that part of the legacy of the father's untimely death was the mother's manifestly denied but repeatedly insinuated blaming of her daughter for his abrupt illness years ago. The mother spontaneously mentioned several times that she had never been bothered by the father's allotment of his time and attention. The daughter seemed to me to be unusually timid and deferential in her mother's presence. However eventually, and after great struggle, she pointed out that despite her mother's repeated spontaneous assertions that there had never been any competition or bad feelings between the two females, that she—smiling tentatively at first as she said this—thought that perhaps there were.

In subsequent individual sessions, this young woman told me that she'd realized why she was always thinking about men in leather jackets. If she were with such a tough man, maybe he'd beat her mother up. Parallels regarding her thoughts about myself and her father began to be explored. Eventually she told me, "I stay sick rather than let out my anger at my mother."

Interestingly, it should be noted that the occasion for these revealing family sessions was her mother's insistence that I fill out forms declaring her daughter to be mentally disabled, so that money could be made available to the daughter from a fund related to the deceased father. The daughter felt more ambivalent about this decision, particularly since being declared disabled would suggest a disqualification of her mental faculties and perspective. There also seemed to be a sense in which another legacy of the father's death would be the concretization of her identity as a "mental patient." But she alternated in saying that she deserved the money. Eventually the mother influenced her daughter to find a different therapist.

Another example will give a picture of "psychotic" communication in finer detail, with another "schizophrenic" client who'd been hospitalized numerous times. This middle aged man told me in his intake session that his previous therapist was a very pushy and provocative man, and described his own similar conflicts with his father. He pointedly declared any discussion of certain other familial issues as being off limits. He next met privately with a psychiatrist to arrange medication. I was later informed that that physician had recommended an injectable major tranquilizer which the client rejected. The psychiatrist acceded reluctantly to the man's request for an oral (pill) form.

However, I didn't know of these things before the first therapy group the man attended, where he immediately remarked on the quietness and the laissez-faire manner in which I conducted the group. This was unlike the "pushy" therapist, he said, who would "make you talk, dragging things out of you, if necessary." He kept interrupting the otherwise relatively quiet group saying, "You're going to pull this out of me anyway, I just know you'll tear it out of me, so I might as well tell you." He then proceeded to tell me about strange occurrences within his brain. He asked if I knew what androgens were. I asked if he meant the hormone. He corrected me, explaining how androgens where when your brain was taken and made into a machine (note the possible play on the word 'androids'). This, he told me, was his basic problem: that his brain was being turned into a machine. He elaborated by referring to the movie *The Stepford Wives*. (That movie was based on the novel of the same name (Levin, 1972) in which a married woman, new to a suburban New England town, gradually discovers that each local housewife is being secretly replaced by a robotic version of herself which will be more servile to her husband. Also, on the day that the protagonist herself eventually succumbs to the forced replacement, she first tries to appeal to a psychiatrist, who instead gives her tranquilizers and suggests that she needs therapy.)

The psychiatrist with whom he had recently met joined the group during this lengthy and excited discourse by this man who was dominating the group with his loud and rambling embellishments of the above noted themes. Gradually, the psychiatrist suggested to the client, gently but indirectly, that perhaps he should have an increase in his medication. When it became clear that the physician was suggesting the medication increase, the man turned to me and asked what I thought. I told him that I saw the issue differently. I pointed out that he'd been talking about powerful doctors, about his expectation of having things torn out of him, and having his brain turned from something human into something machine-like, as well as *The Stepford Wives* imagery. If those were his concerns, perhaps he was saying that tranquilizers, or an increased dosage, weren't what he wanted.

Some weeks later, the same psychiatrist told me that a close relative of this man had written to him requesting that we: (1) insure that the client be declared disabled and get state financial support, and (2) not let him stop taking medications as he'd done in the past when he'd "gone off his rocker," and (3) give the man injectable major tranquilizers in spite of his objection. The psychiatrist told me that he had already written back, acknowledging the letter and generally agreeing with the relative, while pointing out that the client had declined injections. He gave me copies of both letters for filing.

When this man came in for the next group, I told him what I knew of the situation, told him that I hadn't read the letters, but that he was welcome to see them. He read them, smiled, and immediately began to protest that this was a misunderstanding—that he agreed completely with his relative and the psychiatrist, and that he had always agreed to the injectable medication. He preferred it, in fact. He later talked about how his only financial support came from some family members, and that he would just have to wait until they died to get an inheritance. Then he spoke at length about how his mind was being replaced by a machine, and how everything he saw, thought or heard was being broadcast to New Haven. I didn't see the connection until the end of the group when I found a state disability evaluation form in my mail box, sent to me by the man's relative, with a return address in New Haven. After the group, the man remained to receive an injection of major tranquilizers by syringe.

In the next session he attended, this man described a vignette in which he had been sitting, minding his own business and smoking a cigarette, when a person came up to him and threatened him with a knife. He said that the guy who threatened him must be crazy, and the only way to handle such a crazy person was to get out of there. I thought perhaps it was not an accident that he had mentioned his assailant's ethnic background (which was the same as that of the psychiatrist), and that he had spoken of being threatened with a sharp object.

Here is another, more longitudinal description of a therapy. This young woman had been hospitalized previously many times, often with different "psychotic" diagnoses. She spent her first individual session speaking of the fact that people's eyes changed. She asked me if I knew of time shifting, how people could come from the past into the future and vice versa. Primarily she spoke of her telepathic contact with a popular celebrity who had been her childhood lover and therapist. This celebrity often said demeaning things to her, but he had also been the *best* lover. He maintained contact with her now by putting voices into her head. She also told me that her mother was a famous novelist. That was not literally true, but I later learned that the author she named was known for her sexually explicit writings with incestuous overtones, and for some biographical controversy regarding the reality of her own incestuous experiences.

Over some months in therapy she seemed to hint indirectly at her fears about our relationship. As I would wonder out loud about the potential meaning of stories she told me, she would then often speak more directly of her fears that I didn't like her, was bored or angry, or didn't think she merited individual therapy sessions. Many times I felt the issue of my trustworthiness was being raised, particularly whether I would take responsibility for my contribution to some difficulty between us. For instance, once I returned to the clinic office to be told by a secretary that a relative of this woman had called long distance several times in my absence, and was again on the phone now asking to speak with me. I chose to take the call, explaining to the relative that I could say nothing about someone in therapy. I agreed to hear the relative out, with the understanding that I would repeat all that was said to the client later. The relative then criticized my attempts to help the client, telling me that I didn't realize how sick she was and how much more directive involvement she needed.

When I opened the next individual session by relaying this occurrence to the woman, and acknowledging the potential breach in confidentiality in my handling of the situation, she assured me that this was fine and that I could continue to handle such situations in the same way in the future. She then told a vignette about her boyfriend, whom she thought was unfaithful to her. She thought he might have given out the keys to their apartment to someone else. She also said that she thought that their phone was tapped. I pointed out the potential parallel between her vignette and how I had started the session; that my handling of the phone call could be described as a breach or unfaithfulness in a relationship, or the violation of a trust involving a previously secure structure or private conversation. She said nothing at first, but then nodded her head vigorously. We discussed how to handle such situations in the future, with her choosing that I should not accept calls from anyone.

Not long after that, by chance I encountered this woman as we both were swimming in a public pool. I was particularly uncomfortable with this because of her ongoing references to her celebrity therapist/lover. In the following weeks I pointed out her indirect references to relationships in which boundaries were blurred, and in which people were potentially devious, sometimes with sexual overtones. I referred specifically to the swimming pool encounter, and I decided to reiterate the limited and specific nature of our work relationship together.

As our work continued, this woman increasingly hinted at sexual concerns. One afternoon, uncharacteristically, she telephoned me. She sounded very shaken and frightened as she told me that she was "beginning to remember things." She went on to detail how she had been molested as a child by that celebrity, or someone who looked like him. (I had previously noticed that there were two men about whom she would sometimes vacillate in recounting memories, saying it was "either him or someone who looked like him"–the celebrity and her father.) She said that a cuddly stuffed animal toy had been used to violate her sexually. She calmed eventually as we talked, but I was still surprised later in the afternoon when she called me, quite emotionally composed, and told me that those things she had described hadn't happened. She said she had made them up.

At times this woman acceded to family members' requests for family sessions. Guidelines were established making clear that we would only meet at her discretion, and that only she could choose to reveal any material from the individual sessions. With her mother present she began to use imagery of sexual secrets, referring to events that had occurred previously. Eventually, since it appeared that the mother was hinting at her discomfort with the daughter's allusions to sexuality, the daughter seemed to more directly request to discuss sexual incidents that may have occurred when she was a child. The mother looked genuinely chagrined and uncomfortable, but eventually spoke of how school counselors had pointed to possible sexual imagery in pictures her daughter had drawn as a girl. The mother then compellingly spoke at length about her own very rigid upbringing, and the supreme discomfort she felt in discussing sexual matters. She described her sense of being overwhelmed, unprepared and unable to deal with them as a mother years ago. She very tentatively agreed that perhaps there had been sexual occurrences or preoccupations that had troubled her daughter since childhood. The daughter seemed very attuned to her mother's hints at how frightening and threatening she found these topics to be. I was reminded of the times my client had told me that she received government money as a pay-off for her silence, and that she feared she would be killed if she discussed certain topics.

Some weeks later I was notified that this woman had been brought to the emergency room by her family members, who were trying to convince her to be admitted to an inpatient unit. It was the day of her usual session, so I offered for her to keep that appointment if she chose to. She showed up with her family. Family members started out by telling her that she wasn't rational right now, and that she should recognize that she was sick, and that her "schizophrenia" was probably going into phase. She was quiet at first. Eventually she interrupted, yelling about a plot, a conspiracy with the CIA and the FBI involved, and that everyone seemed to be brainwashed and hypnotized. She told me that she thought I was brainwashed too. She then started to hint at sexual intrigues or secrets. When I got her permission to comment on the "plot" and "brainwashed" imagery and the reference to sexual intrigues, I connected these images with the discussion in the last family session. She began to calm a bit. I ended by asking what had happened with that discussion since the last family session. She then yelled, "That's just it! No one will talk to me about it!"

During this session, the family eventually confirmed that when the patient was a girl, some adult sexual infidelities had led to a gory death in the family's presence. Actual death threats at that time, as well as the fear that the courts might still now intervene if other illegalities and sexual misconduct were revealed, made people quite hesitant to speak openly. However, it was eventually revealed that the client was not the only sibling who had confirmed that ongoing secret sexual abuse of children by adults had taken place in the home. At the end of the session, one family member who had been quite verbally abusive and threatening toward me on some occasions, sincerely asked me if I thought that the family might be undermining the therapy.

Here are a few other highly condensed descriptions of what I saw as the central imagery that developed and was explicated in therapy with other "schizophrenic" patients:

A woman felt that for years she had lived within a conspiracy against her in which people wanted her to be sick or die. She wondered if the conspirators wanted her to drink bleach. She was unsure if she'd ever been made to drink urine or to eat worms, and she had a vision of having a group of men sticking a bird down her throat. More than once, as I would sit with my hands together, supporting my head, and with my fingers under my nose, she would exclaim, "Dr. Shulman, why are you jamming your penis up my vagina?" Eventually she began to have memories of having been raped by a group of men, in one instance, and revealed other chaotic and frightening aspects of her sexual history both within and without her family.

A woman who was usually silent in group therapy was provoked and taunted by a male group member of another ethnic group. She began to scream at him that she was a full blooded Sioux Indian (not factually true) and told him that she would take a tomahawk to him and turn him into a squaw, and then dance around inside his tepee and see how he liked it. At a later group she revealed a childhood history of racially tinged rapes.

A teenage girl who dressed revealingly and applied unusually large amounts of makeup spoke very little, but sometimes mentioned visions of snakes crawling into her bedroom at night. Eventually she told of ongoing incest which was corroborated by others.

A woman nervously asked to have her young daughter accompany her to her first appointment with a male therapist. She then spoke of how she had tried to keep Martians out of her room when they hovered by the window, but that they intruded in spite of her closing the window and blinds, and they abducted her. She hesitated, looking at her daughter, but then explained how her captors "examined" her and hurt her in exploring her genital region. She then had her daughter leave the room as we began to explore the possible connections with actual sexual assaults, which she then began to say she had sustained. She also elaborated on a recurring image she had had of male figures who come towards her menacingly. She described how she cries out, but no one hears what she says.

CONCLUSION

Other writers have documented the benefits of similar therapeutic explorations. In *The severed soul,* analyst Herbert Strean (Strean & Freeman, 1990) gives an extended case study to demonstrate the amenability of "psychotic" or "schizophrenic" primary process verbalizations to traditional psychoanalytic exploration (see also Strean & Freeman, 1988). Peter Breggin's *Toxic psychiatry* (1991) gives other similar case examples.

In their book *Psychotherapy of schizophrenia: The treatment of choice* (1981), Karon and VandenBos illustrate through case materials how exploration of such verbalizations provides clues as to their unconscious expression of reactions to trauma and conflict. Others provide similar examples of explorations of metaphors in psychoanalysis or psychotherapy with "schizophrenics" (e.g., Boyer & Giovacchini, 1980; Langs & Searles, 1980; Ferreira, 1960; Karon, 1992; Searles, 1965; Will, 1961). Modrow (1992) recounts in autobiographical detail the compounded tensions in his family and early life which led to his own unusual behaviors and fantasy, earning him the diagnosis "schizophrenic."

Spence (1987) criticizes the tendency toward "narrative smoothing" in most condensed case presentations. I believe his arguments raise important issues. Clearly, the clinical situations I presented here have emphasized certain of the symbolic highlights or recurrent themes in each therapy. The reader sees these events only through my eyes, in condensed form and with hindsight. However, I emphasize that I am not urging clinicians to accept my viewpoint on the subject of metaphorical communication in "psychotic symptoms" solely on the basis of these descriptions. Instead, I urge clinicians to listen to people with such "symptoms" and "diagnoses" in therapy, and to judge my perspective based on their own subsequent experience. Certainly I am trying to be compelling here in recreating the stories of these people's lives. But that is because I have been compelled by these camouflaged communications, which repeatedly seemed to be hinting at traumatic and deeply upsetting experiences. Such seemingly formative and traumatic experiences have come into sharper focus and have regularly been confirmed in reality over the course of discussion in therapy. The strongest argument I can provide that does not depend heavily on the inevitable human appeal, charm and drama of a case description, is to encourage clinicians to try such an exploratory approach in therapy themselves.

I urge clinicians to avoid being blinded or prejudiced by predominant theoretical models which suggest that the temporary incomprehensibility of someone's actions or speech can be resolved by the affixing of labels such as "delusions," "hallucinations," "thought disorders" or "psychoses"; as if those labels explained to us that these phenomena should be deemed (or dismissed as) narratively or symbolically invalid, inexpressive or ultimately incomprehensible. Those models then suggest to clinicians that they should take such clinical phenomena as "symptoms" of a "diseased mind," or evidence of an incompetent person. The "patient" is then seen as someone who should be "helped" by a "supportive," "directive" or semi-paternal or authoritarian relationship. In other words, such temporarily incomprehensible words and actions are taken as a cue or justification for ending therapeutic exploration between two consenting and competent autonomous adults, and for beginning a relationship which is invalidating for the "patient," and which is symbiotically dominant/submissive. Szasz (1976) describes the relationship that typically develops when "schizophrenia" is "treated" as a "disease."

I will conclude by mentioning some writers who offer corollary support for the perspective I have presented. Watzlawick, Beavin and Jackson (1967) state that "psychiatric symptoms" of "schizophrenia," viewed from the standpoint of communication studies, suggest that these symptoms may be viewed as a "reaction to an absurd or untenable communicational context (a reaction that follows, and therefore perpetuates, the rules of such a context) . . . " (p. 47). My repeated observations (such as the cases cited) suggest to me that their viewpoint is relevant and accurate, and contributes to understanding each individual therapeutic puzzle presented to us in clinical practice. Their view also suggests just how powerful it can be to break that cycle of problematic communication.

Rosenberg's (1984) analysis of "psychosis" emphasizes:

> These symptoms of schizophrenia are enormously varied. Some involve thought, some affect, some behavior. There is no obvious logical connection among them. Although they are apt to be characterized by distress and disability, the chief feature that they have in common, we believe, is that naive external observers are unable to understand the response in terms of the actor's frame of reference, intentions, motives, or desires, in ways that fit the observer's theories about the wellsprings of human action. When this occurs, the behavior is viewed as insane. (p. 293)

The author underlines that, for professionals and laymen, the determination of "sanity" or "psychosis" is based on the ability of the observer to understand or "take" the role of the other (the patient), with one exception. People are not judged to be insane "when the observer attributes the failure to take the role of the other to his or her own limitations" (p. 289).

Only after considerable clinical experience with case examples such as those cited did I read Ferenczi's (1932/1949) "Confusion of Tongues . . . " paper. Although such aspects of psychoanalysis were not commonly discussed then, Ferenczi felt that his patients were often critical of him, in a way that was expressed in somewhat veiled communication. When he began to respond to those criticisms, with some acknowledgement of the element of accuracy in their descriptions of his inevitable faults, flaws or mistakes, he found that people were more likely to begin to reveal to him formative traumatic events and patterns in their childhoods. He felt that it was a unique and moving therapeutic event for such people to have a powerful figure acknowledge responsibility for their hurtful contribution to their difficulties. It was on the basis of numerous revelations of trauma by patients in therapy that Ferenczi urged Freud to reconsider the change of position he had taken, in which Freud abandoned his original thesis that emotional difficulties tend to stem from actual trauma (sexual and otherwise), and not from unconscious fantasies. (We have already seen how Lidz /1973/ came to a similar viewpoint.)

It is worth repeating the factors that Ferenczi believed facilitated revelations of both trauma and complicated emotional binds in therapeutic work. He came to focus on camouflaged and ambivalent communication that often suggested a criticism of the therapist. He found that it was a powerful therapeutic intervention to acknowledge the potential relevance of that communication within the therapy, and with special regard to actual actions and comments of the therapist that are, to at least some extent, accurately perceived as injurious or hurtful. For the "psychotic" patient, this also entails acknowledgement of the "meaning in their madness," the relevance of their primary process associations, particularly in the context of the therapeutic situation.

In this regard I am reminded of two quotes. Szasz (1976) said: "Actually, often the only thing 'wrong' (as it were) with the so-called schizophrenic is that he speaks in metaphors unacceptable to his audience, in particular to his psychiatrist" (p. 23). Twenty years previous to that, Bateson, Jackson, Haley and Weakland (1956) had noted, "the peculiarity of the schizophrenic is not that he uses metaphors, but that he uses *unlabeled* metaphors" (p. 253). Later they pointed out: "The convenient thing about a metaphor is that it leaves it up to the therapist . . . to see an accusation in the statement if he chooses, or to ignore it if he chooses" (p. 255).

I urge clinicians to consider doing traditional, consensual, exploratory therapy, that includes reasonable attention and respect for therapeutic frame and boundaries, with the people we call "schizophrenic." Consider the possibility that a metaphorical (or unconscious) commentary is being provided, just as you might listen for it in therapy with others. Let it be your guide. I believe you will be convinced of the poetic relevance of what is being said.

It is possible to do a voluntary, exploratory, uncovering or psychodynamically informed therapy with the people we call "psychotic" or "schizophrenic" that is not so different from therapy with other people. Although the metaphors that are explored at first may seem relatively more unusual, bizarre or somewhat alien; to borrow a phrase from Harry Stack Sullivan, the therapy and the life stories that emerge, nevertheless will be "more human than otherwise."

NOTE

1. Language can both communicate and conceal. Throughout this paper I use quotation marks to demarcate certain commonly used psychiatric terms and concepts that connotatively perpetuate a perspective that I wish to call into question. The quotations serve as a reminder to the reader to question certain problematic assumptions that I believe develop from our uncritical use of those terms.

REFERENCES

American Psychiatric Association. (1987) *Diagnostic and statistical manual of mental disorders*. (3rd ed., rev.). Washington, D.C.: Author.

Andersen, H. C. (1981) "The Emperor's new clothes," in *Michael Hague's favourite Hans Christian Andersen fairy tales*. New York: Holt, Rinehart & Winston.

Bateson, G., Jackson, D., Haley, J. & Weakland J. (1956) Toward a theory of schizophrenia. *Behavioral Science,* (1) 251-264.

Bentall, R., Jackson, H. & Pilgrim, D. (1988) Abandoning the concept of 'schizophrenia': Some implications of validity arguments for psychological research into psychotic phenomena. *British Journal of Clinical Psychology,* (27) 303-324.

Bettelheim, B. (1956) Schizophrenia as a reaction to extreme situations. *American Journal of Orthopsychiatry,* (26) 507-518.

Boyer, L. B. & Giovacchini, P. L. (1980) *Psychoanalytic treatment of schizophrenic, borderline, and characterological disorders*. New York: Aronson.

Boyle, M. (1990) *Schizophrenia: A scientific delusion?* London: Routledge.

Breggin, P. (1983) *Psychiatric drugs: Hazards to the brain*. New York: Springer.

Breggin, P. (1991) *Toxic psychiatry*. New York: St. Martin's Press.

Burrell, M. (1992) 'Schizophrenia' as a strategic concept, not brain disease. Given at American Psychological Association Convention, Washington, DC.

Clinton, J., Sterner, S., Stelmachers, Z. & Ruiz, E. (1987) Haloperidol for sedation of disruptive emergency patients. *Annals of Emergency Medicine,* (16) 319-322.

Cohen, D. (1989) Biological basis of schizophrenia: The evidence reconsidered. *Social Work,* (34) 255-257.

Cohen, D. & Cohen, H. (1986) Biological theories, drug treatments, and schizophrenia: A critical assessment. *The Journal of Mind and Behavior,* (7) 11-36.

Coleman, L. (1984) *The reign of error*. Boston: Beacon Press.

Dohrenwend, B. P. & Egri, G. (1981) Recent stressful life events and episodes of schizophrenia. *Schizophrenia Bulletin,* (7/1) 12-23.

Ferenczi, S. (1949) Confusion of tongues between the adult and the child. *International Journal of Psycho-Analysis,* (30) 225-230.

Ferreira, A. (1960) The semantics and the context of the schizophrenic's language. *Archives of General Psychiatry,* (3) 128-138.

Flack, W. Jr., Miller, D. & Weiner, M., eds. (1991) *What is schizophrenia?* New York: Springer-Verlag.

Grinker, R. R. & Spiegel, J. P. (1945) *Men under stress.* Philadelphia: Blakiston.

Karon, B. and VandenBos, G. (1981) *Psychotherapy of schizophrenia: The treatment of choice.* New York: Aronson.

Karon, B. (1989) "Psychotherapy versus medication for schizophrenia: Empirical comparisons" in *The limits of biological treatments for psychological distress.* Fisher, S. & Greenberg, R., eds. New Jersey: Lawrence Erlbaum.

Karon, B. (1991) Interaction between genetic vulnerability and rearing environment: Discussion of Dr. Pekka Tienari's paper. Given at Xth International Symposium for the Psychotherapy of Schizophrenia, Stockholm, Sweden.

Karon, B. (1992) The fear of understanding schizophrenia. *Psychoanalytic Psychology,* (9) 191-211.

Langs, R. (1976) *The bipersonal field.* New York: Aronson.

Langs, R. & Searles, H. F. (1980) *Intrapsychic and interpersonal dimensions of treatment.* New York: Aronson.

Leff, J. & Vaughn, C. (1980) The interaction of life events and relative's expressed emotion in schizophrenia and depressive neurosis. *British Journal of Psychiatry,* (136) 146-153.

Leifer, R. (1990) Introduction: The medical model as the ideology of the therapeutic state. *The Journal of Mind and Behavior,* (11) 247-258.

Levin, I. (1972) *The Stepford wives.* New York: Random House.

Lidz, T. (1973) *The origin and treatment of schizophrenic disorders.* New York: Basic Books.

Lidz, T. & Blatt, S. (1983) Critiques of Danish-American studies of biological and adoptive relatives of adoptees who became schizophrenic. *American Journal of Psychiatry,* (140) 426-435.

Modrow, J. (1992) *How to become a schizophrenic.* Everett, Washington: Apollyon Press.

Persons, J. B. (1986) The advantages of studying psychological phenomena rather than psychiatric diagnoses. *American Psychologist,* (41/11) 1252-1260.

Putnam, F. W., Guroff, J. J., Silberman, E. K., Barban L. & Post, R. M. (1986) The clinical phenomenology of multiple personality disorder. *Journal of Clinical Psychiatry,* (47) 285-293.

Rappaport, M., Hopkins, H. K., Hall, K., Belleza, T. & Silverman, J. (1978a) Are there schizophrenics for whom drugs may be unnecessary or contraindicated? *International Pharmacopsychiatry,* (13) 100-111.

Rappaport, M. (1978b) "Are drugs more than palliative in the management of schizophrenia?" in Brady, J. P. & Brodie, H. K., eds., *Controversy in psychiatry,* Philadelphia: Saunders & Co.

Rose, S.P. (1984) Disordered molecules and diseased minds. *Journal of Psychiatric Research,* (18/4) 351-360.

Rosenberg, M. (1985) A symbolic interactionist view of psychosis. *Journal of Health and Social Behavior,* (25) 289-302.

Sarbin, T. R. & Mancuso, J. C. (1980) *Schizophrenia: Medical diagnosis or moral verdict?* New York: Pergamon Press.

Sarbin, T. R. (1986) "The narrative as a root metaphor for psychology" in *Narrative Psychology,* Sarbin, T. R., editor, New York: Praeger.

Sarbin, T. R. (1990) Toward the obsolescence of the schizophrenia hypothesis. *The Journal of Mind and Behavior,* (11) 259-284.

Sarbin, T. R. (1992) "The social construction of schizophrenia" in *What is schizophrenia?* Flack, W. F., Miller, D. R. & Weiner, M., eds., New York: Springer-Verlag.

Sass, L. (1992) *Madness and modernism.* New York: Basic Books.

Searles, H. F. (1965) "The differentiation between concrete and metaphorical thinking in the recovering schizophrenic patient," in *Collected papers on schizophrenia and related subjects.* New York: International Universities Press.

Searles, H. F. (1975a) "The patient as therapist to his analyst," in *Tactics and techniques in psychoanalytic therapy. Vol. II: Countertransference.* Giovacchini, P., editor, New York: Jason Aronson.

Searles, H. F. (1975b) "Countertransference and theoretical model," in *Psychotherapy of schizophrenia,* Gunderson, J. G. & Mosher, L. R., eds., New York: Aronson.

Siegel, R. K. (1984) Hostage Hallucinations. *The Journal of Nervous and Mental Disease,* (172) 264-272.

Spence, D. (1987) *The Freudian metaphor.* New York: Norton.

Strean, H. S. & Freeman, L. (1988) *Behind the couch.* New York: Wiley.

Strean, H. S. & Freeman, L. (1990) *The severed soul.* New York: St. Martin's Press.

Szasz, T. (1965) *The ethics of psychoanalysis.* New York: Delta Books.

Szasz, T. (1976) *Schizophrenia: The sacred symbol of psychiatry.* New York: Basic Books.

Szasz, T. (1987) *Insanity: The idea and its consequences.* New York: Wiley.

Watzlawick, P., Beaven, J. H. & Jackson, D. D. (1967) *Pragmatics of human communication.* New York: Norton.

Will, O. A. (1961) "Process, psychotherapy and schizophrenia" in *Psychotherapy in the psychoses,* Burton, A., editor, New York: Basic Books.

Surviving the "Mental Health" System with Co-Counseling

Janet Foner

SUMMARY. The writer describes reclaiming her life after institutionalization with emphasis on the importance of Re-evaluation Counseling (RC). She describes her earlier hospital experiences and how she came to reevaluate them. Case studies with the positive impact of RC also are examined, as is the author's current emotional situation. *[Article copies available from The Haworth Document Delivery Service: 1-800-342-9678.]*

In 1967 I was a senior painting major in college, terrified at the prospect of being on my own with no likely job or husband to provide income. I took risks to help the situation and felt both powerful and scared, crying and shaking and telling my friends how to change their lives.

One night I never noticed that I didn't go to bed, as I was writing to my ex-boyfriend in metaphors. A friend who was worried about me came to

Janet Foner, MPSSc, is the International Liberation Reference Person for "Mental Health" System Survivors in the Re-evaluation Counseling Communities; Co-Coordinator, Support Coalition International; and Director, Leadership Exchange Listening. Mailing address: 920 Brandt Ave., New Cumberland, PA 17070.

Author note: I've used quotation marks around all "mental health" terms which refer to the medical model, including "mental health" itself, because these terms are inaccurate and untrue in my opinion. I have used them because they are the terms with which most people are familiar that refer to the concepts I am talking about.

[Haworth co-indexing entry note]: "Surviving the 'Mental Health' System with Co-Counseling." Foner, Janet. Co-published simultaneously in *The Psychotherapy Patient* (The Haworth Press, Inc.) Vol. 9, No. 3/4, 1996, pp. 107-123; and *Psychosocial Approaches to Deeply Disturbed Persons* (eds: Peter R. Breggin, and E. Mark Stern) The Haworth Press, Inc., 1996, pp. 107-123. Single or multiple copies of this article are available from The Haworth Document Delivery Service [1-800-342-9678, 9:00 a.m. - 5:00 p.m. (EST)].

see me. I told her she shouldn't be engaged to her fiance because she was marrying him to please her family and he wasn't right for her. (She did marry him and got a divorce about seven years later.) I wasn't communicating very clearly. She got scared and called my mother, who took me to the school psychologist, the family doctor, and finally the outpatient clinic of the local psychiatric hospital. I was very angry at my mother for insisting I go in the hospital; we often had angry arguments. I knew a lot about mental hospitals, having just studied abnormal psychology in school. I was also getting in touch with my feelings about growing up as a Jewish woman and having to live with sexism and anti-Semitism combined, not to mention the economic oppression of artists. Not able to put all this into words at the time, I knew something was very wrong with our society. Since I identified with blacks, due to my hair being similar to theirs, I screamed at the doctor on hospital admissions about how racism is wrong, in metaphors. What I was trying to say was that since the two unusual colors of my mother's coat, orange and green, could harmonize, why couldn't blacks and whites?

Unfortunately, the doctor didn't understand and called for a nurse and two attendants to take me to a locked ward. With no discussion, no questions asked, and no reading of my rights they dragged me upstairs. While I tried to fight them off, they injected me with a huge amount of thorazine and put me in seclusion for about nine hours. It was like an incomprehensible nightmare. I felt I would die or jump out the window, but the only window was very tiny and barred, so I did neither. Later I thought I heard voices in the radiator, voices talking about or to me on the radio, saw a picture of a lion coming out of the newspaper, and thought I was going to be electrocuted both by the floors in the hospital and by the hairdryer in the hospital beauty shop. These experiences were diagnosed as "psychotic." My exact diagnosis probably was "paranoid schizophrenia." I spent a lot of time with nurses, attendants, other patients, psychiatrists, the dance therapist, talking, crying, and shaking a lot about my experiences. Unknowingly, that helped me. Psychologists tested me many times to determine why I recovered from "psychosis" so quickly, but didn't find the answer.

Ten months after my entry into the hospital I was released, feeling that my life was over at age 22. I was in much worse shape than when I entered the hospital. I was afraid to go out of the house, certain that people knew I was an ex-"mental patient" just by looking at me and were talking about me, was sure no one would hire me though I'd finished school shortly after my release, felt very depressed and hopeless, and had no idea what to do with my life. Gradually, with the help of family and friends and my psychiatrist (who slowly took me off thorazine over a period of about eight months), I got back on my shaky feet, got married and moved out of state to start a new life. The year 1970 was the last time I ever sought or received help of any kind from the "mental health" system.

By 1973 I was back in my home state, taught art at a local community art center, painted, and cared for my 1 and 1/2 year old son. I looked fine to others but felt very bad about myself inside, was painfully shy, got depressed very frequently, had few friends, could not talk about my experiences as a "mental patient," and still didn't know what I wanted to do with my life. I also was scared about raising a child.

Through a friend, I got involved in Re-evaluation Counseling (also called Co-Counseling), an international network of people from all walks of life, age groups, races and cultures who exchange peer support in a natural self-healing process. The purpose is to recover full use of one's intelligence in order to improve one's life on all levels, and ultimately the lives of one's friends, family, and co-workers. A leadership development community to foster social change, it encourages people to think about, develop policy on, and take action against all oppressions and to teach others to use the process to aid in building liberation movements. When I read the theory of Co-Counseling I was immediately struck by its clear explanation of a mystery to the "mental health" field: What was happening to me when I was hospitalized? How had I recovered from the experiences that led to my hospitalization?

The theory suggests that all people are by nature zestful, loving, cooperative, creative, and, unless they have damage to the forebrain, completely intelligent. We also have the capacity to heal ourselves from emotional and physical damage through an internal process outwardly indicated by tears, laughter, trembling, sweat, angry sounds and movements (not to be confused with destruction of property or violence towards someone), animated, non-repetitive talking, and yawns. Infants intuitively seek attention in order to heal themselves via the above methods of discharge from difficulties encountered before or during birth. Older babies are gradually socialized to control and suppress their healing process.

It is hypothesized that people ordinarily take in information through the senses and store it in usable form in their brains. When people get hurt, they stop thinking momentarily (a "state of shock") and the information from the hurt experience comes in through the senses and is mis-stored in non-usable form. If the person gets a chance to release emotion in the above ways until the self-healing process is completed, the information from the hurt experience will be re-evaluated and stored in usable form. However, most of us, except as young infants and sometimes not even then, don't get to do that. We are prevented from doing so by the adults taking care of us, all of whom were socialized at an early age by those taking care of them, in the same way. Some adults try to comfort babies, hush them, distract them, believing that emotional discharge is the hurt itself, rather than the healing of the hurt. Other adults, lacking time or attention, may verbally abuse a baby (as in "Shut up or I'll give you something to cry about!"), or may ignore a baby's cries. In one way or another the baby or young child is forced to hold back the discharge/re-evaluation healing process, since babies depend on their adult caretakers for survival.

As the child gets older, more and more hurts occur and are not healed or are only partly healed. Each person develops rigid behavior patterns coming from the particular ways the person got hurt and couldn't heal. People do not use flexible intelligence to respond to the current situation. Instead, they are influenced by past hurts, do not think clearly, behave in ways harmful to themselves or others, do not act or feel like the creative, joyous persons they are, by nature. We think and behave rigidly in many ways, called "patterns," which often obscure our true nature.

The socialized prohibition of the natural healing process has a great deal to do with the functioning of the "mental health" system. Applying the above theory to the commonly held beliefs about "mental health," in the above view everyone is hurt to one degree or another and virtually no one has had a chance to recover completely. Thus, everyone has difficulties in functioning well since there is no dividing line between the "mentally healthy" and the "mentally ill." It's all relative, and relative to the situation. There are "acceptable" distress patterns, such as smoking, social drinking, amassing nuclear weapons, adults yelling at children. These will not get one labeled "psychotic," but staying in bed all day and not going to work or believing something is real that doesn't appear that way to others may get one so labeled. These distresses are designated symptoms of "mental illness" but are not any more indicative of something wrong than the first set of distresses mentioned, the "acceptable" ones.

"MENTAL ILLNESS"

There are generally three kinds of phenomena that get called "mental illness": One is the discharge process of healing. *The Diagnostic and Statistic Manual* that psychiatrists use is filled with descriptions of "symptoms" of "diseases" such as crying extensively, trembling, sweating, "laughing inappropriately." What is known as a "nervous breakdown" is not the nerves, but the rigid patterns breaking down that have controlled and held back discharge and healing for years. The patterns are breaking down and allowing the person to heal, but our society is focused on making money and not on healing. It doesn't ordinarily allow for times and places to heal. Adults are expected to go to work and produce; thus it appears inappropriate for adults to stop everything in order to heal. The same is true of children once they reach school age.

A second kind of phenomenon usually called "mental illness" is actually the person intuitively seeking attention to heal by displaying a "pattern," a recording of a past hurt in the person's behavior, in hopes that someone will notice and help.

The third kind of phenomenon is often the reason for children and teens being labeled "mentally ill" when they behave in a way that, usually unawarely, attempts to enable another person to discharge and heal. This type of behavior is often misunderstood and not seen as the often desperate attempt that it is to correct an intolerable situation for that person by getting the adult in charge or a close person to discharge, re-evaluate, and change the situation.

With this framework, hallucinations can be seen as the attempt by one's body to draw one's own attention to distresses (often-forgotten ones) that very much need to be discharged in order to continue to survive. People whose discharge processes have become extremely inhibited and who also have enormous amounts of hurts accumulated apparently can reach a saturation point where the body takes over and tries to preserve itself. Delusions can be seen as a literal replay of a piece of a past hurtful experience or a confusion of a past hurt with a present situation. The person talks about it as if it were going on now in an attempt to discharge and re-evaluate it. With the use of the natural healing process, hallucinations and delusions will disappear as the person discharges and re-evaluates.

CONTINUING A STORY

While I haven't completely discharged and re-evaluated my own story, I have re-evaluated and have figured out the following. I had grown up believing I was ugly and could not attract men. This came mostly from anti-Semitism, growing up in a society where the blond, blue-eyed, voluptuous Marilyn Monroe-types are the ideal; the stereotype of a Jew, dark-skinned, with dark, curly hair and a large nose, is an unacceptable way to look. I look like that stereotype as well as not being voluptuous and was seen as unattractive by my family and the Jews I went to high school with (95% of the school). They had internalized the anti-Semitic viewpoints, as

I had. Also, Jewish women are considered to be asexual compared to Christian women, and so I thought myself incapable of attracting men.

As a young woman, I was to marry and raise children, according to what I'd been told. When I lost the only boyfriend I'd ever had, someone I wanted to marry very much, in the fall of 1966, I felt awful. However, after a week of crying, I decided to change my life and go out and meet men. Previously I had been a very shy recluse. In April of 1967, I went out with three different men, all tall, dark and handsome by society's standards and very interested in me, all in the same week.

I had not cried enough about losing my boyfriend and grief began to resurface, once I saw that I couldn't be that unattractive if these attractive men were interested in me. I became very confused and terrified because this was a complete turnaround to how I had previously viewed and lived my life. At the same time, I felt hope for the first time in seeing my dreams could be realized. Everything was happening too fast for me to take it in, including my fast-approaching graduation. If I were living in a healing-oriented society, it would have been recognized that I was going through profound emotional changes connected with new understandings about myself, life, relationships with men, and the oppressions in society. Not yet understanding it all, I spoke in metaphors that more directly expressed what was not yet clear to me in linear thinking. In the language of Re-evaluation Counseling (RC), events had provided a contradiction to my distress patterns. I could see that they were not the reality, which allowed me to begin discharging and getting rid of my patterns. Unfortunately this natural process was interrupted by my stay in the hospital and the thorazine I was forced to take there.

In Co-Counseling sessions I began discharging the grief about losing my boyfriend and did so for several years. I began to look at how sexism and anti-Semitism had affected my life and then attempted to act like the beautiful Jewish woman I am, and discharged the emotion arising from doing same. Taking that direction led me to make positive changes in my outward appearance, to seek new friends who were not depressed and who could support me well, to become close to many people, to take leadership within RC and form close counseling relationships with several men who knew I was beautiful and could counsel me well on that issue. Gradually I stopped being shy, lost most of my fear of men, became a well-known leader in RC and later in the ex-"patients" movement outside of RC. I began to write well, became much more self-confident, able to speak in front of groups, and to see myself sometimes as beautiful.

One day I looked in the mirror and saw a most beautiful, joyous, alive, sexual, self-confident, happy woman and knew that it was the real me, the person I'd lost touch with, during very early distressing experiences from which I'd never had a chance to recover. This was the same woman I'd been looking for when I was in the hospital and had to ask one of my friends there who I was. She had said to look in the mirror, which was very helpful, but it wasn't until 1985 that I could see there what I really had needed to see all along. Since that day in 1985, I have never again doubted my beauty or lost sight of who I really am. Now I can always look in the mirror and see a beautiful woman and can make friends with any woman, no matter how her looks are viewed by society; I am no longer jealous of other women or wish to be someone else. I have many close friends, both males and females, and am self-confident most of the time. What I was trying to heal in 1967 has been healed completely, although I still have other things to heal.

EXPERIENCING THE HOSPITAL

The other main re-evaluation I have done about my "mental health" story concerns my hospital experiences. When I got out of the hospital I had been "brainwashed" into believing that I was a "deeply disturbed person," that my hospitalization had helped me tremendously in my recovery through all-powerful psychiatrists' help which had saved my life, that I had nothing much to do with my recovery, but the psychotropic drugs I took really helped me and I needed them since there was something very wrong with me. I had believed this last most of my life, but my hospital experience intensified and made "official" that belief. It is only in recent years, after talking about and discharging extensively on my hospital experiences, that I realized how damaging those experiences were. I could then stop blaming myself for what happened to me and recognize that the shame I felt about myself as an ex-"mental patient" was coming at me from societal oppression. It had no foundation in what was true about me, since there really was nothing wrong with me, i.e., I had no permanent emotional defects. While I had never enjoyed my hospitalization, I believed it had been good for me, or at least that it was the only way to help me, given my condition.

In recent years I have realized how damaging being put in seclusion twice was to me. Those two experiences left me feeling extremely terrified and unsafe. My ability to stand up for myself, to seek to fulfill my goals, to speak rather than being very quiet were all badly damaged. In recent Co-Counseling sessions I am at last able to discharge terror and grief from being locked in seclusion. For many years it was too hard and too terrifying to even talk about it at all, let alone feel and discharge how it had felt.

I now am able to talk about seclusion in public speaking engagements or other advocacy situations and to be less quiet, less scared. I am also more able to believe in my ability to take charge of situations and fulfill my goals.

When I was first forced to take psychotropic drugs I knew they made me feel awful, exhausted, lethargic. But by the time I left the hospital, I'd been told so much that they were good for me that I believed it. At that time, feeling numb seemed better than feeling terrified. Later, as I regained more ability to discharge and to feel more alive, aware, and also to just feel more, period, feeling numb seemed the worst of the possibilities. It became clear to me that the drugs I was forced to take had kept me from the discharging I needed to do at the time and had given me extra damage that needed to be healed—two years of my life where I barely felt alive.

As I learned to Co-Counsel, I began to realize that the psychiatrists I'd had, while somewhat helpful in that they listened well and did not try to discourage me from discharging, had not really "saved my life." Their analyses of me had only increased my shyness, shame, and belief in my own permanent "defects." The natural healing processes which I and everyone else have, were what had "saved my life." I was and am in charge of my own process. In recent years I have realized that I was never in need of hospitalization (nor do I believe anyone else is, unless they need surgery or other types of medical care for identifiable physical ailments) and that what I really needed at the time were some RC sessions and a few other kinds of support.

I have also realized that when I thought the other patients were plotting against me and when I thought that, on leaving the hospital, people on the bus were talking about me, I felt that way due to distress experiences of the past. As a child I had been scapegoated in a number of groups. When I felt as unsafe as I did in the hospital, I unawarely felt as I had as a child, since being forced to live in a group situation with strangers reminded me unconsciously of those past times.

When I thought I was going to be electrocuted, it was because I was born in 1945, right around the time U.S. citizens heard about the Holocaust, the bomb dropped on Hiroshima, and my father was still recovering from almost dying and was now paralyzed permanently from the waist down. While still in the womb, I am sure I felt my mother's fear of all this and also became frightened. I'm convinced that I was born terrified into a family in severe crisis. I must have assumed that I was always in danger of being killed as I was born while so many people were dying. I identified the hospital with a concentration camp because the hospital staff could not be trusted; they said they were helping you and then force-drugged you and locked you in seclusion, a euphemism for solitary confinement.

All of this combined to make me believe I was going to be killed, just as the Jews were told they were going to the "showers"–which turned out to be the gas chambers. Thus my fear of the beauty parlor was that the hair dryer could really be an electroshock machine (which I'd never seen, but knew were used on other patients on my ward). Also, I'd been terrified as a child by movie and television stories about prisoners being electrocuted– and there I was, locked up and definitely a prisoner. When I figured out, in recent years, why I feared electrocution in 1967, it all made sense and I no longer thought of my fears as strange, or proving I'd been really "crazy."

In general, re-evaluation of all the above has allowed me to feel equal, on a par with other leaders, not unfit to talk to them as I had felt before. I am able to talk easily about my "mental health" experiences both publicly and privately, or not talk about them without feeling like I'm hiding something. Previously I couldn't talk about this subject even to close friends. I am now proud to be a psychiatric survivor. It feels good and powerful to be a leader in "mental health" system change, no longer ashamed of my experiences in the system.

RE-EVALUATION COUNSELING (RC)

What was helpful to me when I was in the hospital turns out to be exactly the natural healing process we call RC. If this process is done formally, two people agree to exchange an equal amount of time giving each other attention, often an hour each. The two people, for the first hour, are focused on the process of one person's reemergence (uncovering the person's inherently good nature where it has been obscured by patterns and living on the basis of that nature) and what will allow that person to think, decide, and act outside of patterns and to discharge the patterns.

The roles are reversed for the second hour with focus on the second person's reemergence. Each is in charge of the session from his or her point of view. If the person in the role of client finds that the person in the role of counselor is not being helpful, not paying attention, or is thinking about the counselor's own distress, the client may stop the session and counsel the counselor until able to return to that role. The client always decides what to bring up in the session, given the current capabilities of the counselor and the depth of discharge and distress that the client is currently able to deal with. In this way, trust and safety are built up gradually and deeper and deeper levels of discharge and distress are reached. The client tries out the counselor's suggestions before deciding, due to distress, not to use them, although if the counselor's suggestion is truly on the mark, the client will begin to discharge without having time to debate about it.

The counselor thinks about the client independently of him/her. The client will often say one thing and really mean another; the counselor must rely on intuition, keen observation, knowledge of the person, knowledge of basic theory, and testing out what works to be able to be effective. The counselor is constantly learning to counsel better, becoming more and more aware of what is or isn't promoting the client's reemergence. The two are engaged in a give-and-take interaction on both sides and truly working cooperatively together, using each other's thinking. The counselor never analyzes or gives advice to the client.

The goal of the process is always to seek re-emergence, including the elimination of patterns through discharge. Understanding what happened to cause the patterns is never a goal or an end-point; it may be a beginning for some of the work and is usually a by-product of it. There are no rigid techniques, although there are some general guidelines. A maxim is that the best technique is the one you invent at that moment. For the process to work at its best, it is always helpful to do fresh thinking as you go along. Practical ideas for ways of working are exchanged among Co-Counselors, but these must be adapted and changed as they are used in order to be workable. Flexibility, and paying complete, aware, loving attention are the main skills needed by the counselor. Since we as human beings are all natural counselors and clients of this sort, these skills are not really learned but reclaimed.

During the session the client usually will begin with a description of positive recent events in order to pull attention away from distress enough to be able to have the slack needed to bring up old hurts. The first task in the session is to focus attention fully on the current moment and the benign general nature of reality. A good deal of time may be spent this way, sometimes the whole session. Then the client will bring up any minor problems and perhaps spend 10-15 minutes talking, laughing, etc., about these. Next the client will state the goal of the session—such as setting goals for life changes desired, counseling on what has come up while trying to reach previous goals, continuing to work on an area defined in previous sessions. The counselor will remind the client of how he/she acted before being conditioned and in all ways possible provide for the client a view outside of the patterns currently being tackled, and any others that come up in the process. As the client begins to discharge, the counselor will encourage that process and provide attention to allow the client to better be able to think about his/her reemergence. The goal is never to adjust to any situation that is not working well but to regain the ability to flexibly handle any problem and change situations so that they work well for the client.

At the end of the agreed-upon time, the counselor will ask the client questions to draw attention off of the distress brought up in session onto pleasant and interesting things in the current environment. Then or in a later, separate session counselor and client switch roles. Thus the healing process never becomes one of a person assumed to be "well" "fixing" someone who is "sick." Mutual respect, lack of hierarchy, and true empowerment become possible. A real cooperation between a counselor and client, a real pulling for each other on an equal basis, becomes possible.

I have used this process with many Co-Counselors who are psychiatric survivors like me, all once diagnosed "psychotic" but now no longer using the "mental health" system or psychiatric drugs, as well as with many current and former "patients" who are not Co-Counselors but have learned something about the process from me. All of these people have been able to improve their lives by using the Co-Counseling process and many have used the process to recover from the effects of hospitalization, psychotropic drugs, electroshock (as far as possible given its possibility of at least some permanent brain damage), and other mistreatment within the system. They have also healed from experiences for which they were hospitalized, such as hallucinations and delusions. Many have used the process to recover from the effects of and fight the oppression of "mental patients," eliminating their own negative feelings about themselves coming from societal stigma, for example. The following stories about some of these people (using pseudonyms) are used with their permission.

PEOPLE WHO HAVE USED THE PROCESS

Michael was hospitalized in 1976 after he stopped eating, moving, and talking. He felt like dying, was starving himself to death and was having a number of very vivid hallucinations. Soon after hospitalization he began talking again and was released in the custody of his parents (he had been living on his own prior to that) with the provision that he take large doses of Haldol and see a psychiatrist as an "outpatient." He was doing this when his closest friend, a Co-Counselor, came to visit. Adam asked Michael what was going on; Michael began to cry profusely as Adam listened. Later Michael visited Adam for several weeks and learned to Co-Counsel from Adam and some of his friends. He cried a great deal in many sessions for a year or two. During that time he moved to his own apartment and later to a house with friends, stopped taking the Haldol and stopped seeing his psychiatrist. He used many sessions to counsel about the effects of the Haldol on him, and to discharge the negative effects of institutionalization and therapy. He also used many sessions to discharge about his hallucinations and remembered the occluded incident that was the basis for most of them.

The hallucinations included seeing his sister dead (she was and is alive) and seeing Jesus in many forms. Michael remembered that when he was three his sister, who was one, had almost drowned. His mother had left him home alone and asked him to pray for his sister to live while she took her to the hospital. Michael was a very religious child and felt it was his responsibility to save his sister, to whom he was very attached. He felt that God had answered his prayer when she did recover, and that he had a special and powerful relationship to God because of that. As a little boy, terrified that his sister would die and grief-stricken about that, he was left alone and never helped with these feelings. It wasn't even acknowledged that he might have feelings about his sister almost dying since as a boy, he was not supposed to cry or show fear. Many years later, the woman he had planned to marry married someone else. Shortly after that Michael's lover had an abortion of their baby, which he wanted her to have, but was not able to tell her. Michael was not able to cry about either of these losses, both of which were very hard to accept. Sometime after that he began wanting to die and seeing the hallucinations about his sister and Jesus, including one in which Jesus seemed to rip open Michael's heart.

As he was seeing the hallucinations, Michael cried and shook a lot and did more of the same in later sessions on the hallucinations. After he remembered the occluded incident about his sister, he corroborated the story with his mother, saw the connections between the early near-loss and the later losses and began to change his life to be able to live outside the patterns he had acquired from those hurts. To be able to deal with major griefs without discharging them he had spent about two years on marijuana and other street drugs; he eliminated that addiction from his life. He had dropped out of college after losing his first love and didn't know what to do with his life. He lived close to a poverty existence on part-time jobs. To do something about "mental health" oppression, he got involved in the ex-"patients" liberation movement, started a political action group of psychiatric survivors and began writing about our liberation. Michael went back to college and graduated and started his own successful business. He is now a leader in "mental health" liberation as well as an admired expert in his second, new business venture.

I met the man I'll call Robert in 1984 at his first RC workshop. He was extremely shy, had little self-confidence and rarely spoke in a group. He had been court-committed to a forensic institution for the criminally "insane" because he had been charged with trespassing and had previously seen a psychiatrist. He was judged incompetent to stand trial and was locked up for eight months. This hospitalization was so painful that he would have committed suicide but couldn't figure out how to do it there. A therapist he later worked with stopped seeing him because he had so much difficulty releasing his anger. At the RC workshop, a man I'll call Cal was counseling Robert and asked him to pretend Cal was an attendant who was going to take him away to the mental institution. Cal took Robert's arm and asked Robert to pull away from him saying "No! I won't go!" loudly; Robert was thus able to discharge a great deal of anger.

Robert continued to discharge anger, grief, and shame about his hospitalization and began to make changes in his life. He had a high-paying, professional job but was not happy in it and so decided to quit, live on savings, and work in the ex-"patients" movement, with the plan of eventually getting a paying job in the movement. He became president of his state's survivors' organization, was appointed to a number of state and county "mental health" boards, became influential there, and was asked to speak at various conferences. Robert also became certified to teach RC and his support group of RC psychiatric survivors grew from two to eight. No longer very shy, he is increasingly self-confident and effective as a leader, and is now becoming influential as a national leader in the survivors' movement. Robert is very rarely held back by angry feelings or feeling suicidal.

I've known Rachel for about eight years. When I first met her she was very quiet, sometimes got severe headaches when trying to deal with her feelings, could not think of herself positively or as a leader. She saw herself as needing help and incapable of giving much to others. She had received a series of about 30 electroshocks during several hospitalizations. In counseling she discharged a lot of terror and grief about her hospital experiences as well as many negative feelings about herself. Rachel started to speak up more, began giving parties, became more outgoing and fun loving and became certified as an RC teacher. This meant taking on leadership and thinking of herself as a leader. She doesn't get headaches as often now and sees herself as capable and as having something to offer.

Alice had a son labeled "hyperactive" and "learning disabled" and was told he might have become "schizophrenic" if he had not been brought in to see the therapist. She was told by her therapist to consider her husband her fourth child (besides her actual three children) because he would not take responsibility in the marriage or with the children. Her family physician had given her a number of psychiatric drugs and said she was in "breakdown syndrome" and implied she would be hospitalized if it weren't for the children. Feeling she could not cope with her life, she went into therapy and then got a divorce. Introduced to RC by a friend, she then decided the therapy she was receiving was not useful and left it. Alice also stopped taking the drugs that had been prescribed. She used the RC process in continuing to raise her sons as a single parent and eventually got them involved in it also. The labeled son completed high school and a year of college in which he got A's and B's; he then decided to pursue a non-college career. He just got married in what looks to be a very good marriage for him.

When I met Alice she was very concerned about her son's "mental health" experience and could not deal with her own devastating experience. Through Co-Counseling she began to see how important it was to deal with how she had been hurt by this experience, particularly in not being able to trust her own thinking. Alice discharged a lot about the prescribed drugs and her feelings while taking them and started to re-evaluate her lifestyle. She was struggling to make ends meet in a low-paying sales job, not trusting herself to do what she really wanted to do. She took courses in a type of bodywork and began to combine her ability to do emotional healing work with body healing work and is now seeing private clients. Eventually she will open a full-time business with a partner. Much happier in her new career, she's re-learning to take care of herself as well as others. She also identified herself publicly as a survivor, and discharged a lot of fear while doing so. Alice has been active in a survivors' organization outside of RC and has taken leadership on the issue within RC.

There are many other stories like these, many I know and don't know. I am sure there are a number of psychiatric survivors in RC who don't get in touch with our survivors' network for fear of losing their jobs if they become known as survivors or for other similar reasons. A few more identify themselves each year as we do this liberation work. Much is also being discovered within RC theory and practice about how to focus attention off distress permanently; how to act on one's clear, forward-moving decisions rather than out of distress; how to maintain a reemergent direction in one's life and not sink into distress over long periods of time; how to make liberation movements work well; what to do when someone is in an emotional crisis. This last area is of much interest to psychiatric survivors.

An RC friend of mine, Alan, was at a workshop with a friend of his, Don, who stayed up all night several nights in a row and was feeling so anxious and upset that he could not calm down. Returning home from the workshop, some of Don's friends wanted to hospitalize him. Alan, a psychiatric survivor, knew that Don would not get what he needed in a mental hospital and wanted him to avoid the stigma of being hospitalized. He insisted that he not be hospitalized and not be given psychiatric drugs. Alan stayed with Don for a day, remaining calmly sure that Don was fine and would/could "come out of it," and discussing pleasant and interesting topics. Don was able to regain his ability to sleep, to stop feeling unbearably anxious, and to resume everyday activities without any psychiatric interventions.

Another aspect of this work within the RC community is weekend workshops I and several others have led for people affected by "mental health" oppression. In some, for all RC people, we have dealt with liberation from conformity, often reinforced by mental health oppression. For mental health system survivors, (people who were hospitalized, those who had therapy, and relatives of both groups, mostly children of survivors), we have met separately and together and have worked on bridging gaps between each of the groups. Relatives have also held their own workshops. For the last three years I have led separate workshops for ex-psychiatric inmates. At the first one we spent many hours telling parts of our hospital experiences and putting it all on a chart. We then had a mock awards ceremony for the "best" in each category, such as longest stay or most times hospitalized. The warmth, fellowship and spirited laughter that permeated those events was a true healing time for all of us. At the most recent of these, many people took responsibility for seeing that the workshop went well. This was a wonderful contrast to the way most people envision us to be. When I began doing this liberation work, I had internalized so much "mental health" oppression that I thought I didn't want to meet other psychiatric survivors and that doing such work was painful and would drag one down because of other people's painful stories. In fact, I found the opposite to be true and have never met so many wonderful people or had so much fun as I have in doing this work. At our workshops everyone gets included, those who know each other and those who don't. There is a great sense of ease and well-being. Saturday night is usually skit night where each support group (we divide into small groups around various issues part of the time) develops a skit that satirizes the negative aspects of the "mental health" system or challenges our thinking in related areas. Most of these evenings are spent laughing from start to finish.

In the last few years I've begun to teach RC to ex- and current "mental patients" and "mental health" workers outside of the RC communities. While I have not as yet done much long-term work with these people, most have been very enthusiastic on receiving just a taste of the theory and practice. One group, after practicing methods of appreciating each other, decided to do an appreciation day on their own, using the skills I'd briefly taught them, and had each person in their drop-in center be appreciated by the whole group. A woman who attended an introductory one-hour session of RC that I gave at a conference went home and led an all-day session for her state-wide "mental health consumer" group using the skills she learned.

At a leaders' training session I worked with one of the leaders in an RC counseling session. I basically told him how good he is and what a good leader he is, but was not sure how useful the session was to him since he did not discharge very much at the time. Months later he mentioned the counseling I had given him at a meeting we were both attending. He said it was very helpful for him and got him out of feeling depressed. He said he thought more people should get a chance to do this. People who have attended introductory workshops on RC at conferences ask me to do Co-Counseling with them at later conferences, call me for the same reason or ask me to lead longer workshops for their self-help groups. People are eager to regain these skills once they glimpse the possibilities. It gives people a lot of hope. One woman told me that her friend, who attended an RC workshop I did at a conference, had tried everything to get help for years and this was the only thing he'd found that was helpful.

In the past year I've taught a series of day-long, monthly workshops for a group of psychiatric survivor leaders, about half currently "outpatients" in the "mental health" system. One of these people now plans to teach a similar series for people she works with (she's an ex-"patient" mental health worker). Another said this course kept him from being rehospitalized during a crisis. Another person who couldn't speak in public has now become an advocate. One man has used the process to stop his periodic depressions. All have begun to regain their abilities to heal themselves.

To find out more about RC, contact Harvey Jackins, the International Reference Person for the RC Communities, at 719 Second Ave. North, Seattle WA 98109, USA; Telephone 206-284-0311. For further information on the psychiatric survivors' movement in RC or on workshops for your survivors' group or "mental health" agency, contact the author, Janet Foner, at Leadership Exchange Listening, 920 Brandt Ave., New Cumberland, PA 17070, USA; Telephone 717-774-6465. (For information about Support Coalition International, a national human rights coalition for alternatives to psychiatric oppression, open to the public, contact the author at same address.) For writings by psychiatric survivors in RC about our experiences in the system and changing it, write Rational Island Publishers at P.O. Box 2081, Main Office Station, Seattle, WA 98111, USA. Ask for *Recovery and Reemergence #3* (partly by "mental health" workers and partly by survivors; includes the first draft liberation policy statement for "mental health" system survivors–$2 plus postage) and #4 (all by survivors, with second policy statement–$3 plus postage). The revised version of the second policy statement can be ordered for $3 plus postage as a pamphlet called "What's Wrong with the Mental Health System and What Can Be Done About It."

Yielding to a Higher Power

Louis Birner

SUMMARY. People caught in the agony of addiction and the grip of psychosis need to find new ways of coping with the demands of reality and staying alive. This chapter deals with the struggles of a patient who is a manic depressive, was addicted to alcohol, other drugs and food. Keeping him alive and separating him from his submissive attitudes, psychotic past and suicidal behavior was the treatment challenge. Such patients must learn to use the therapeutic situation to claim their own power. They must give up the need to die mentally and physically. To win the battle against the psychotic process and the addictive defense both therapist and patient need to find the courage to look at past traumas. They then must be creative enough to find new ways of living out life in the present. Even the most disturbed of people can grow emotionally as a new understanding of self and reality emerges in the treatment process. The psychotic past finally becomes a thing past. *[Article copies available from The Haworth Document Delivery Service: 1-800-342-9678.]*

Will is a piano player/singer/entertainer at a fancy East Side bar in New York City. His analyst-to-be walked into said bar one night and ordered a glass or two of orange juice as he listened to Will play and sing. Amazed to see anyone at the bar order orange juice, Will asked me about this and

Louis Birner, PhD, is a member of the National Psychological Association for Psychoanalysis and the American Psychological Association. He is in the private practice of psychoanalysis, psychotherapy, and group therapy. He has done research and published in the areas of the resistances to the creative process and the psychological aspects of procrastination, betrayal and addiction. Mailing address: 50 East 72nd Street, New York, NY 10021.

[Haworth co-indexing entry note]: "Yielding to a Higher Power." Birner, Louis. Co-published simultaneously in *The Psychotherapy Patient* (The Haworth Press, Inc.) Vol. 9, No. 3/4, 1996, pp. 125-140; and: *Psychosocial Approaches to Deeply Disturbed Persons* (eds: Peter R. Breggin, and E. Mark Stern) The Haworth Press, Inc., 1996, pp. 125-140. Single or multiple copies of this article are available from The Haworth Document Delivery Service [1-800-342-9678, 9:00 a.m. - 5:00 p.m. (EST)].

125

seemed struck dumb when I said I never drank. This was especially significant because Will was a chronic drinker. Whenever I visited the bar Will
cut his act short so he could spend a few minutes talking with the "local
shrink."

Will's appearance presented a contradiction. Handsomely and tastefully
dressed, a man full of charm and wit who sang and played beautifully, he
was at the same time a hundred pounds overweight. As he worked through
the night, he would drink hard liquor mixed with soda and yet never
appear drunk. The management gave him his drinks for free, and Will
would order them two or three at a time. When they were consumed, he
would dramatically tell the bartender that there were "dead soldiers" on
his piano and he needed replacements. As an entertainer, he never seemed
tired or in a bad mood. Rather, his affect was expansive and elated and this
hyperemotional tone gave his performances an extra bounce of spirit. He
came across as an "up guy" who could belt out a song with gusto. He was
never dull. Another feature of his talents worth noting is that he had a vast
repertoire and knowledge of modern music. His speaking voice gave the
impression of an educated cultivated person who read extensively.

During one of his breaks Will informed me that he'd like to talk to me
outside. His tone was quite serious. Once outside, he related that he was
quite worried about his health. Sometimes he felt depressed. His doctor
said he was prediabetic; this was very dangerous because he was 100 pounds
overweight. When I agreed that he could be in serious trouble, Will
laughed and said, "Do you know what I have in my safety-deposit box? A
hundred Seconals and a bottle of Remy Martin. If I have to go out, I go out
in style."

His grandiosity, denial, and self-destructive attitude rendered me impotent and I responded, "Will, there has to be a better way." My remark seemed
to have no effect.

A few weeks later Will asked me for my card. He said he was worried
about his weight and about his son. Inasmuch as I had some personal
relationship with him, I declined to see him as a patient and referred him to
another analyst. A few days later Will called to say that he had seen the
"Shrink" but that there was no chemistry between them and that he would
really like an appointment. It was obvious to me that this was a man who
pounded out his mania on a piano and sedated his moods with alcohol.
Will was a manic depressive, manic with an alcoholic defense, eating and
drinking himself to death.

Will's first session was a monument to his defense of denial. Arriving
on time, he discussed his problems in a theatrical way. He was aware of his
drinking and of being overweight and was not too happy about it. Yet he

showed no real concern or anxiety over his plight. In short, he was putting on a rehearsed and polished performance. To go along with his exhibitionism and narcissism would have been a disservice to him. He wanted sympathy, but in no way did he seem eager to do anything positive about his problems. He had started drinking in his teens and never stopped. He had seen weight doctor after weight doctor and had never really lost an ounce. He was an obese alcoholic with a prediabetic condition. Time was running out for him.

During the first half of his session I said nothing other than to ask a question or two. Finally I asked, "Do you think you have any real problems?"

Amazingly enough, he answered in a light, pleasant tone, "Not really. I have always been able to cope."

I realized that if he was to be helped, his massive denial and pleasant composure would have to be punctured. I responded by saying, "Will, I have heard a lot of bullshit in my time, but you, you stupid bastard, take first prize. You are 100 pounds overweight. You are almost a diabetic. Once you get diabetes and mix it with alcohol, you stand an excellent chance of losing limbs. Tell me, how would you like to be a one-armed piano player or walk around on stumps? That's something that would really make your son feel good? You are 6 months away from being dead. If you want to see me, you are going to have to do two things: One, see a doctor and get on a diet and have your blood checked; and two, join Alcoholics Anonymous. If you are not ready to meet these conditions, let's end the session now."

Will was struck dumb, amazed at my toughness and frankness. Immediately, something happened. He saw that he was given a task: lose weight and stop drinking. He also chose to start to idealize me and made a submissive gesture, saying, "You are the doctor. I agree to do what you say."

The rules of treatment were outlined, and Will began therapy on a once-a-week basis. Treatment can be defined as having two phases: The first phase could be called "the dry run"; the second phase can be considered "the real thing." It is of particular note that the first phase of treatment was punctuated by what Will called a "manic attack." This occurred one night after work when he fell off a chair and seemed to lose emotional control over himself. He went to a mental hospital and had himself committed for the weekend. No doubt he went into a panic state. After the weekend he felt fine. At that time, Will attached no major significance to his attack and, despite my probing, the true meaning of the "attack" was not apparent. Not then.

The first year of treatment had an educational flavor to it. The goals of maintaining his contact with A.A. and with his medical doctor were frequently reinforced. Because he had idealized me, it was very easy for Will to "follow orders." As a result, two significant and gratifying events occurred. He gave up alcohol completely and lost 100 pounds in the first 3 months of treatment. In doing this, he illustrated the execution of two needs often found in the personality constellation of the manic depressive: challenge and triumph. It is through challenge and triumph that the depressive can avoid a sense of despair (Fenichel, 1949).

As is the case with most people who are very disturbed, Will was highly undersocialized, lacking self-loving and self-protective judgment. His reality sense was tenuous, to say the least. The early focus of therapy centered on life management. This was in keeping with meeting maturational needs and reducing his toxic interactions with life. Transferentially, he saw me as his glorified advisor and a narcissistic extension of himself. He presented the following very damaging behavioral problems:

1. Scoring pills for his girlfriend.
2. Involvement in shady deals:
   a. buying stolen property,
   b. lending money.
3. Involvement with dangerous and exploiting women.
4. Stealing from women's pocketbooks.

Will's self-damaging behavior was seen as a need to create situations that produced humiliation or the threat of humiliation. He wanted to risk provoking authority, especially in those circumstances that could lead to punishment. There is no doubt that authority represented the maternal authority figure of the past. He would narcissistically overvalue his girlfriend and then submit to her wishes through a projected idealization. The marvelous lady had to be pleased. He would risk arrest by buying pills for her illegally. Stealing from other women and seeking out abusive women appeared to serve only one need: to risk humiliation and punishment.

Will was shocked, amazed, and gratified when I told him, "You are a humiliation addict and it appears that you need a daily fix."

"God dammit," he responded, "you are right. Thank you."

The issue of self-worth and giving up humiliation was an important treatment focus. When he spoke about wanting to do self-damaging acts, he was given minor humiliations by being called an idiot or a schmuck. These toxoidal interventions served to provide an answer to his quest for abuse and humiliation, yet at the same time worked to reduce his actual self-destructive behavior. Will was encouraged to develop appropriate relationships and a stable design for living. He was seen on a once-weekly basis for a year. During that time no dreams or childhood memories were forthcoming. Then he said that financial problems made it impossible for him to continue. He praised me in glowing terms and was pleased with what he had accomplished in a year. Indeed, he was right. He did give up his alcoholism and he did lose 100 pounds. Quite a year's work! When Will left treatment, he had completed his dry run in therapy. He had yet to face the massive conflicts that plagued his life; he had yet to confront his childhood amnesia. One can conjecture that his leaving treatment was a way of saying that he could not integrate any more success into his life. Success and the manic-depressive state do not mix very well.

About a year later, Will called to say that he would like to resume treatment. On his arrival, I noted that he had put on a bit of weight. He was as expansive as ever, speaking in high and eloquently grandiose tones. A.A. was still an important part of his life, but trouble was brewing within him because he could not master the fourth step of his alcoholism treatment program.

"Just what is the fourth step?" I inquired.

"It is 'yielding to a higher power,'" he responded.

Will made a very interesting Freudian slip when he said that the fourth step was "yielding to a higher power." In reality, A.A.'s fourth step is "a fearless and searching moral inventory of ourselves." No doubt this confusion can be seen as his trying to deny his own guilt and severe superego pain. The only "moral inventory" he was given in his childhood was one of self-hate. His next statement clarified why he feared a fearless and searching moral inventory. "Also there is something else I have to tell you. I never told you the truth about my childhood. There is a lot I remember but have been too ashamed to tell you."

A contract was formed with Will: He would use therapy to work on the fourth step and to fill in the history of the childhood that he worked so hard to conceal during the first year of his treatment. What follows here is a condensation of many sessions. His resistance to bringing in the material can be fully understood because his childhood reeked of humiliation, horror, alcoholism, incest, psychosis, and filth.

Will's telling the truth about his childhood can be seen as maturational. Quite often, though, he did not want to speak about it. He was given negative support by being told such things as, "Of course you had the worst childhood in the world," or "No doubt you are a horrible person, but tell me about your loving family." These toxoidal interventions helped Will to speak about his past.

Of particular interest is the story of his maternal grandparents. The grandfather was the scion of a rich distinguished Protestant family. The grandmother was a poor shanty-Irish Catholic. She became pregnant out of wedlock and, much to their families' consternation, they married. The grandfather was a professional man who, a few years after his marriage, fell from a great height and became a hopeless cripple confined to a wheelchair.

Will's mother's history is quite sketchy. She grew up in a home with an invalid father and an alcoholic mother. She showed talent in music and dance at an early age and was considered a great beauty. She managed to become one of the famous showgirls of her day. A rather rich and influential man seduced her and made her pregnant. She elected to have the child and recapitulated her mother's role, with the exception of not marrying the man who impregnated her. Both mother and child lived in the home of the maternal grandmother. It was the time of the great economic depression of the thirties. Will came from a family of money and did not suffer financially during this chaotic period. Indeed, he was to become a "rich child."

Grandmother now had a captive family at her disposal. Will's mother, Belle, became grandmother's drinking companion. In a short time she lost her beauty and became a chronic alcoholic. Although the house was large, she wound up sleeping in her mother's bed. Alcohol use was daily—either at home or in bars. When drunk, they vomited and defecated in random spots in the house and made little effort to clean things up.

There was a sober period to the family day: between waking up and some later hour in the afternoon, when the drinking started. Drunk or sober, grandmother ruled the house with a sadistic iron hand and also a very neglectful one. Will and grandfather were almost uncared for. Grandfather could void in his pants and not be attended to for days. Mealtime consisted of supper, which was not good in terms of the quality of the food and horrible in terms of the quality of the social interaction. Will was there to be insulted or ignored.

The family structure consisted of an evil alcoholic woman dominating a broken-down crippled husband, a degenerating daughter, and a psychologically scarred grandson. The pathos of this scene was enormous: a rich, promising professional wrecked, drunk, and in a wheelchair; a beautiful talented showgirl becoming fat and alcoholic; and a grandson forming an identification with disaster.

Will's earliest childhood memories consisted of his wandering down the street of his small town alone. He recalled making ketchup sandwiches for himself because no adult was there to make breakfast. He was neglected, abused, or ridiculed in the family interactions. Sometimes, as is the way with alcoholic people, he received avalanches of affection, only to later face subsequent indifference. To confuse and to add an even stranger irony to his existence, Will discovered a huge cache of money in the basement. He would walk around his town as a rich kid buying favor and friendship, trying to compensate for his emotional poverty.

It is significant that there were no benign or consistently loving figures in his childhood. Education meant little to him. He functioned inconsistently in school and did poorly in athletics. His childhood existence was one of loneliness and isolation. Showpeople occasionally came to the family home; Will observed them and became a self-taught actor. As a youngster he also learned to play the piano by ear. His late childhood and early adolescent years were punctuated by his doing periods of time in a series of torturesome boarding schools. Theatrical and musical interests were the only light in his dark and unhappy childhood.

Two very traumatic events occurred during Will's adolescence. His grandfather died, and he had to call the police; mother and grandmother were out drinking at some bar. Will felt enormous shame bringing the police into the vomit-filled, shit-filled house. The second event was even more traumatic. When he was 14, Will's grandmother took him to bed with her and seduced him. The grandmother also slept in the same bed with his mother. It appears that this woman, on a conscious and psychotic level, lived to incestuously destroy everyone about her. As a result of his grandmother's action, Will was never interested in developing an active and fulfilling sexual life. Rather, his sexuality has been mixed with humiliation and indifference. All of his life he has walled himself off from any appropriately loving involvement with the opposite sex.

Grandmother died when Will was 18. Her estate was a monument to her life of destructiveness. The family home was such a filthy wreck that it was barely saleable. His mother had degenerated into a fat alcoholic. The once-famous beautiful showgirl was to end her life working as a chambermaid in a low-class hotel. Will was already an alcoholic. Although grandmother was dead and buried, she lived on in her grandson's psyche, urging him on to alcoholism and self-destruction.

Will related that grandmother had great contempt for men and loved the company of women. Indeed, she slept with and was sexually involved with her daughter. She was a hateful anti-Semite and treated everyone else like dirt. What is most is most interesting is that Will's memory of her abusing him is very limited. Psychic crimes were committed against him; however, other than the incestuous experience, his memory is quite blank. This repression is probably at the core of his manic-depressive posture. What was repressed was probably the destruction of his sense of value and self-esteem. He was also robbed of his right to be angry. The higher power that Will always yielded to was his mother and grandmother. Astoundingly enough, he has no remembrance at all of his mother. One could speculate that both mother and grandmother were merged into one traumatic image. The image deprived him on an oedipal level of any true feeling of worth and self-satisfaction. A sense of trust or comfort was lost in the dawning of his life. No doubt he experienced depression and rage in his earliest years.

After the death of his grandmother, Will tried a number of jobs. When he was not working he was drinking. As fate would have it, he wandered into a bar one night, saw a piano, and started to play and sing. Quite by accident, he found a career for himself that met his alcoholic, musical, and exhibitionistic needs. One can conjecture that his alcoholism was a way of dealing with his mania. Drinking slowed him down; it stabilized his moods; and it also destroyed him physically and mentally. Perhaps on some deeper level, when he was playing and singing in a bar, he was reunited with his childhood family—only this time he was accepted and beloved. Like his family, he was also quite drunk.

Will's psychosexual history can be marked by one word: abuse. He has no memory of his first 5 years. Early feeding and toilet training must have been emotional disasters. This devastation can be seen as reflected in his food and alcohol addictions. It is noteworthy that Will always wears a strong cologne. The smell of the shit and the vomit of his childhood haunts him. He makes his contact with the world through exhibitionism and manic affect, not through intimacy.

Will's marriage was part of a fantasy and was very brief. He wanted to marry a Protestant American type of woman and have a son to whom he could give the best so that the boy could climb the ladder of success. By a strange quirk of fate, he met a woman who went along with this need and they produced a son. After a year or two, Will left his wife and son, Bob. He has been devoted to them both all his life. True to Will's fantasy, Bob graduated from a prestigious college and became a professional, marrying a woman who came from a good background. In deference to his grandmother, Will created another matriarchy. Unlike his grandmother, however, he genuinely cared for his son. Like his father, Bob drinks; however, his drinking is situational and occurs as he nears periods of success.

After leaving his wife, Will met the girlfriend who was to be the passion and disaster of his existence. Roberta was extremely beautiful. She was also a pillhead and a prostitute. Her life was punctuated by periods of imprisonment for drug use. Will "mothered" her; he fed her, gave her money, and supported her habit by scoring pills for her. Scoring pills is dangerous because it involves risking arrest and/or being mugged. If arrested, Will could have lost his license and his vocation.

Roberta and Will had an interesting sexual pattern. Neither was interested in sexual intercourse per se but any style of oral stimulation was a delight to them. "Going down" on Roberta was the ultimate thrill for Will and gave him endless sexual pleasure. Roberta was never around for long. Her being arrested or finding other men interfered with their relationship, and she both exploited and humiliated Will during their time together. True to his childhood history, Will mixed sex and humiliation. Indeed, during his fourth year of treatment, Roberta died of an overdose in his bed, leaving a pile of vomit. In deference to her memory, Will bought a tombstone for the lady.

Interestingly enough, Will related that he never had any homosexual contacts. With women, he tends to be sporadic and impulsive. His penis means little to him, his partner means little to him. His main source of gratification is his mouth. Like most people who are locked in psychotic conflict, he is fixated at the oral level of development. Like the infant, he can feel both elated and starved emotionally with great ease.

Shortly after Will started treatment for the second time, he found a new weight doctor who, among other things, prescribed the drug Elavil. As a result Will became quite manic. I suggested he consult a psychiatrist about whether or not he should be on Elavil. After the consultation with the psychiatrist, he was placed on lithium, which tended to stabilize him.

When Will returned to treatment, he stated that he really wanted to get into his analysis. He wanted to know if there was anything he should do as a patient. I suggested that any information about his childhood would be helpful. Much of Will's treatment has centered on his childhood remembrances.

Will's degree of repression is remarkable. His mother never existed in his recollections. In 5 years he has not brought in one dream. Childhood loneliness and abuse are the two most significant communications. Memories cluster only about grandmother. He vaguely describes his mother as his protector against his grandmother. He tended to cast her in the role of his protector and friend. No doubt this was a reaction formation to the rage he feels toward his mother. Repression and the absence of memories point to an extreme depressive posture in his early childhood. The more of his awareness and cognition he could wall off, the safer he felt in the grim and traumatic days of his early development. His preoedipal emotions probably center on the loss of love from and his rage toward the maternal introject. Early acts of separation and individuation were not supported inasmuch as the mother herself was a dependent alcoholic who was narcissistically involved in her own destruction.

In the transference, I am somewhat idealized. One of the things that makes treatment most meaningful to Will is that it is a situation where he receives no abuse. In terms of his ego functioning, he seems to need caring but cannot take too much friendliness or warmth. He is the exhibitor, actor, performer. The analyst is the listener. In fact, one of the things I do is help him get his act together. Will likes toughness. His manipulativeness and need to delude himself are challenged in treatment. In one session he acknowledged, "I am glad I cannot bullshit you."

Will's elation, charm, and up mood can create in the therapist a positive countertransference on a subjective level. Such positive countertransference reactions must be looked on with suspicion. Will's idealization, warm mood, and fund of stories only serve to cloud his depression and self-destructiveness. To reward the charm and the elation in any way is a disservice to him and to the treatment. On an objective countertransference level, Will's praise, warmth, and idealization must be seen as a treatment resistance. This resistance is to be challenged as it serves to distance him from making emotional contact. In Will's case this idealization seemed a mask of hatred inasmuch as none of the principals of his childhood stimulated a true feeling of love and caring.

It is important to note that, like most psychotics, Will has a problem staying in reality. At work he does fine. An elated manic can have a soothing effect in a bar full of mostly depressed people. Many customers have praised him for his ability to lift them out of their depression with his music and the warmth of his personality. It's after work that Will is in trouble. Unless he has a routine, he falls apart. He can be an avid reader, a many-mile walker, or an engaging talker. It is when he feels he has nothing to do that his anxiety level rises, heightening his potential to overeat or even to drink. His friends are few and often have their own addictive problems. Will feels he needs challenges; these challenges help keep him reality bound. Without appropriate and consistent stimulation he can regress into a depressive, depersonalized state.

On some levels, Will transfers his babyhood into treatment. He wants an approving mother; he needs limitations, support, and guidance. In short, he sees his analyst as the mother and father he never had. He refers to me as his "professional." It seems most probable that his reverential feelings are the displaced hope of finding a good and loving mother. Will's rage has only one outlet and direction—his fury at his grandmother. It also seems likely that this rage is kept under close control; he cannot afford to lose any love objects. This, of course, is the dilemma of the psychotic: the need to hold on to the toxic introjects and the fear of losing them or of displeasing them. Without his work and routine Will falls apart. Vacations are impossible; being out of therapy for a week is most difficult.

Time has a peculiar meaning for Will. He exists in the prolonged battle of his early childhood. The vital emotional supplies of caring, affection, and recognition are only to be found in his audience, his therapist, and a few friends. He is constantly fighting his depression and trying to separate from his hateful introjects.

"THE MANIC ATTACK"

The session before Will's "manic attack" was unusual. He asked permission to bring his grandmother's perfume and to smell it during the session. Perhaps he thought that this would help him to remember. In a theatrical way, he presented the bottle, opened it, smelled it, and put some perfume on his tie. For all of his drama and for all of the pungency of the perfume, nothing happened. No memories of childhood or grandmother were forthcoming. Indeed, this session left Will feeling somewhat disappointed.

Within a week he fell into what he has called a "manic attack." On Sunday he felt a sense of panic and tried to get himself committed, without any success. He called me and his psychiatrist, and he ran to a mental hospital and sat in the emergency room. After the attack, he was a changed person. His voice was slow and heavy; his movements reflected psychomotor retardation; he was confused, emotionally flat, and time disoriented. He appeared drug addicted. He was by no means suffering from mania but was experiencing a psychotic depressive reaction, one that reflected the core of hopelessness of his psyche. Grandmother's perfume brought not only the smells of childhood back to him, but also the major emotional loss of his life. Freud (1917/1957) felt that depression represented a libidinal investment in an unloving object. The unloving object—mother/grandmother—also represents his incorporated object. Will's stuporous depression was a reunion with his introjected family. This depressive mood was in sharp contrast to his joyous and happy mood—which attempted to deny the existence of these introjects and to affirm his own ego. His catatonic-like stupor represents his infancy when he sought after and tried to incorporate a loveless and cruel mother/grandmother figure. A lifelong pathological feeding process, as it were, had been initiated. Feeding at the unbeloved and poisonous breast is a core problem in all depression. When one introjects the unbeloved mother, depression can be seen as an attempt to kill off the self and the introjected object. According to Lewin (1961), the mother can be introjected as both a superego object and an ego object. Disassociative depression is a way of yielding to this mother's dreadful influence and to her hollow, empty breast. In depression, Will yields to her higher negative power.

It took Will 6 weeks to gather enough control over himself to resume functioning. His only activity during this depressive reaction was work, which consisted of playing and singing for 4 hours daily. After work he either slept or ate. He could not remember appointments. Indeed, even when appointment times were written down for him he would not remember to show up. If he was late only one minute, I phoned him. He would then rush over and have a part of his session. This time disorientation was probably a repetition of the way his childhood time was made a chaotic and frustrating stream of events without any rhythm or meaning. His early feeding was most likely an inconsistent and masochistic experience; he was probably fed when mother was sober (which may not have been very often). There was probably no rhythm or pattern to his childhood rearing; consequently, he resisted the pattern of his appointments.

The problem of treating the depressive side of the manic personality is one of not yielding to induced feelings. Gross hopelessness, disorientation, poor reality testing, and a depersonalized form of contact were transferred to me. Will tried to stimulate feelings of pity and frustration in me. It seemed most probable that his depression was covering up a murderous rage toward both mother and grandmother. The challenge of working through a severe depression is one of giving the patient appropriate communication.

I became gruff and unfriendly during this depressive period. This is in keeping with Edith Jacobson's (1971) notion that the severely depressed person cannot integrate warmth or caring. The poison of his depression was fed back to him in a toxoidal way, to reduce his self-hatred. His flat empty state was countered by some very powerful emotions on my part. This is in keeping with Spotnitz's (1985) notion that, when appropriate, the therapist should provide emotions that are missing in the patient's personality. I told him that he was a "goddam schmuck living to please your grandmother by becoming her Zombie," or I made other comments such as, "Don't be an asshole. Stop worshipping that cunt."

Gradually, Will started to remember his appointments. His voice pattern changed; the very heavy tone and slur pattern left his speech. The issue of routine and managing his life came back into therapeutic focus and he was able to work through his depression.

As a means of counteracting his depersonalized depressive reaction, Will occasionally makes plans about his future, plans that often reflect his manic grandiosity, preoedipal states, and psychosexual conflicts. An example of this is his planning a new piano act with a dwarf: "The dwarf will play the part of an aggressive macho male. I'll be the female. We will have purple lights. I'll put false keys on the piano. They will fly off at the right moment. The act will be a sensation."

Role confusion and a need to change sexual roles resulting from his lack of male identity is obvious. The keys flying off his piano may represent his expectancy of castration. Although this "act" gives all the power to the dwarf who is the symbolic mother or grandmother, Will sees this performance as a means of esteeming himself and advancing his career. He does not realize what his symbolically giving up his maleness could mean and means in terms of repeating his childhood and the reexperiencing of his castration fears.

Another "great act" Will is considering is a "Frankie and Johnnie" routine. Frankie is a prostitute, and Johnnie is her pimp. "I'll have her pull a gun and kill me. It will go over great."

Once again, Will is symbolically destroyed by the maternal figure. This fantasy is a denial of the feeling of annihilation and destruction that was so much a part of his early development and the psychic key to his depression.

Hopefully, in time, Will will be able to regulate his life so that he can integrate enough self-esteem to hold his mania and his depression in balance. His need for triumph (his mania) and the sense of defeat (his depression) serve to keep him out of reality and to rob him of a sense of inner peace.

At this point, Will has worked through some of his depression and is somewhat in control of himself. When yielding to the higher power–his mother/grandmother–he is immobilized in depression and loss of reality. In struggling to claim his own ego, he begins to make contact with the world.

THEORETICAL AND TREATMENT CONSIDERATIONS

Therapy has effected some inner psychic change in Will. Five years of once-weekly treatment has regulated his life. Treatment has been most successful in the area of making psychic substitutions. Food and alcohol have been renounced for the triumph of diet and sobriety. It must be noted that these "triumphs" are a very common reaction to a morbid state of depression. The manic depressive is ambivalent toward his own ego. In depression, he is powerless. In mania, which is the other side of his depression, he is triumphant and no longer feels that he has to be afraid. The superego has merged with the ego. In giving up obesity and alcoholism, Will triumphs over mother/grandmother and gives up his morbid identification with them and with his pathological incorporation of them. Mother and grandmother are temporarily destroyed.

Freud (1913/1958) discussed the manic-depressive cycle in his *Totem and Taboo*. He considers the manic-depressive cycle to be a period of increased and decreased guilt feelings, a cycle between annihilation and omnipotence, of punishment and a new deed. In the last analysis, this goes back to the original life cycle of hunger and satiety in the infant. Will's mania can be seen as a reaction formation to his depression, not a genuine "triumph."

What is interesting clinically is that Will also denies and reacts against his depression through exhibitionism. He delights in his weight loss and sobriety and is ready to show and tell the world about it. His exhibitionism is not, however, a measure of an increase in self-esteem. It is a defense against his depression and a way of handling sexual impulses.

In treatment, such patients are basically inaccessible when either manic or depressive. They are often ambivalent and narcissistic and offer great resistance to the analytic process. Two factors are of the greatest help: (a) some enforced stabilization (through medication, treatment, or a life situation), and (b) the free interval (that period in time when neither the mania nor the depression predominates).

Will has experienced both factors in treatment. He does work, and his moods are medically regulated and balanced. There have been free intervals in his analysis. Indeed, he has functioned for 5 years. In his infantile way, he genuinely likes and cares for me, his therapist. The therapeutic goal of working for free periods has met with some measured success. The desired result in the treatment of manic-depressive psychosis is to extend and to make the free interval a major part of the patient's existence. Cases have been noted in the literature where this goal has been achieved. For instance, Abraham (1953, pp. 418-476) succeeded in curing patients afflicted with manic-depressive psychosis.

As many writers have pointed out, depression represents a fixation at the oral level of psychosexual development. The manic depressive is an extreme case of this. Lewin (1950) notes in his concept of the "oral triad" that the sense of elation represents a liberation from profound superego pressures. Elation is a false emotion and serves to deny certain psychic expectancies such as annihilation, castration, incest, and primal scenes. To eat, to be eaten, and to sleep are the baby's earliest psychic expectancies. In the manic depressive, any of these expectancies are tinged with the threat of annihilation.

What is interesting about his case is that it reflects the cyclothymic personality and the pattern of neurotic depression in general. Neurotics do go through swings of mood and use the mechanism of denial. They can also be narcissistic and inaccessible to treatment. However, the problem of treatment is most complicated because we are dealing with psychotic states and preoedipal communications and affects. The critical issues of separation and individuation from early toxic introjects are primary. Giving up the unbeloved breast and incorporating self-loving objects and experiences are necessary in the treatment of both the neurotic and the psychotic.

The work of Spotnitz (1985) has been of particular help in conceptually understanding Will's psychotic communication. Before the therapist can enable maturational changes, he or she must understand the preverbal communications and puncture the narcissist's defenses that make the patient inaccessible to treatment. Both the mania and the depression must be seen as pre-ego feelings. Also, when Will expressed both sides of his psychosis, the therapist had to note that he did not exist for him as an object (human being); rather, if he did exist for Will he was more of an audience. The idealized "professional" was more a psychotic projection than a flesh-and-blood human being.

Part of the process of maturing the patient was to use support to get him to make such valuable contacts as A.A., along with establishing routines of walking and visiting museums and attending musical events. Through treatment Will was–like the toddler–being given permission to walk down the street and to experience life. Discussions of A.A., museums, and concerts had a contact function and were object oriented. His previous alcoholism had kept Will drugged and out of life. His depression was narcotized by his drinking. The depression also represented the preverbal feelings of annihilation that he must have experienced from his drunken mother's inconsistent care. The mania itself can be seen as a total narcissistic involvement, making him inaccessible to contact and treatment.

Fenichel (1945) notes that there are three special difficulties in dealing with the manic depressive:

1. The oral fixation (crucial preoedipal material).
2. The narcissistic nature of the illness and the looseness of the transference.
3. The inaccessibility to analytic influence due to the absence of a reasonable ego.

Working with the narcissistic transference, then, is the best hope of establishing contact. Using a clear period when the ego can be reasonable and in contact with reality is most beneficial.

Emphasis must be placed on dealing with the patient's narcissism in such ways as to help him or her to make emotional contact and to grow up. This is often a frustrating task and a negative countertransference is easily developed and must be fought against as therapy progresses The patient is understood best as a psychotic infant resisting the language of health. Extreme patience and an inner hopefulness are essential in working with such patients. One must seek ways of substituting a reality sense in place of morbid psychotic states and affects.

At the core of the manic depressive is the expectancy of both psychic and physical destruction. Denial serves to keep all morbid expectancies intact. The therapist must work to bring the patient into a reality state free from the torment of introjects. As Will said in one session, "I am getting my hand off the worship button. I feel better."

REFERENCES

Abraham, K. (1953). *Selected papers on psychoanalysis.* New York: Basic Books.

Fenichel, O. (1945). *The psychoanalytic theory of neurosis.* New York: Norton.

Freud, S. (1955). Totem and taboo. In J. Strachey (Ed. and Trans.), *The standard edition of the complete psychological works of Sigmund Freud* (Vol. 13, pp. 1-164). London: The Hogarth Press. (Original work published 1913)

Freud, S. (1957). Mourning and melancholia. In J. Strachey (Ed. and Trans.), *The standard edition of the complete psychological works of Sigmund Freud* (Vol. 14, pp. 237-160). London: The Hogarth Press. (Original work published 1917)

Jacobson, E. (1971). *Depression.* New York: International Universities Press.

Lewin, B. D. (1950). *Psychoanalysis of elation.* New York: Norton.

Spotnitz, H. (1976). *Psychotherapy of preoedipal conditions.* New York: Jason Aronson.

Spotnitz, H. (1985). *Modern psychoanalysis of the schizophrenic patient* (2nd ed.). New York: Human Sciences Press.

No Place Like Home

Robert F. Morgan

SUMMARY. This is a case history, with a 23 year span, of a hospitalized artist's fear of psychosis, treatment, and eventual outcome. Using what would eventually be thought of as paradoxic intention, psychotherapy, and art therapy, the initial year of counseling and discharge are illustrated by examples of the artist's work. The long-term outcomes, expected and unexpected, give a longitudinal perspective in a Hawaiian context. *[Article copies available from The Haworth Document Delivery Service: 1-800-342-9678.]*

PROLOGUE

I owe much; I have nothing; the rest I leave to the poor.

(Francois Rabelais, 1533)

It had been 23 years since his discharge from my care. The voice was mature, relaxed with a stronger island accent than I remembered. "Yes," he said, "I definitely still want you to tell my story. And of course with my art. That's still what I do. Be sure particularly use the name on my canvas: Gordius."

Robert F. Morgan, PhD, is in private practice at 855 La Playa #358, San Francisco, CA 94121-3252.

[Haworth co-indexing entry note]: "No Place Like Home." Morgan, Robert F. Co-published simultaneously in *The Psychotherapy Patient* (The Haworth Press, Inc.) Vol. 9, No. 3/4, 1996, pp. 141-183; and: *Psychosocial Approaches to Deeply Disturbed Persons* (eds: Peter R. Breggin, and E. Mark Stern) The Haworth Press, Inc., 1996, pp. 141-183. Single or multiple copies of this article are available from The Haworth Document Delivery Service [1-800-342-9678, 9:00 a.m. - 5:00 p.m. (EST)].

GORDIUS

The Law of Raspberry Jam: the wider any culture is spread, the thinner it gets.

(Alvin Toffler, 1985)

Hawaii's Portuguese community violated Toffler's law as long as it could. Fifty years ago the jam was successfully thick.

The Portuguese followed the Chinese and Japanese as seduced waves of ethnic workers for the plantations of island entrepreneurs. To keep grounded in their origins, tradition was jealously protected and family expectations were clear.

The Portuguese were World War II "Okies," lured to the island with promise of paradise and exploited in the fields and canning plants by their sponsors. The work was brutal and unrelenting. Into this tropical trap came a young Portuguese family: mother, father, three sons.

The father and his older brother had died of heart failure and exhaustion before Gordius was old enough for public school.

Once he headed for New York to be an actor. Mother wrote him regularly on the impossible odds against this happening. She told him he was free to live his life as he wished but she would probably not survive alone. He was guilty, frightened and unsuccessful. Doling out equal portions of blame for himself and for his mother, he returned home.

He went to the University of Texas—not the most benign environment in that decade for a gay Roman Catholic raised in Hawaii. (Neither of course was New York: his ambivalence at leaving home was regularly reflected in the odds he set against himself.) Again mother wrote dire predictions and guilt-inducing pleas. And again he returned.

Paying more attention to his clear preference for the company of men, he applied to an order of Catholic brothers within the Portuguese community. They told him there was no room for homosexual priests in their order. He swore he would respect celibacy but they were unrelenting. He called them unchristian and was evicted.

The next year he chose better, enlisting in the army. The military, even today, is clearly a great career choice for those preferring the company of their own gender. Gordius thrived, working his way up the ranks to sergeant in four years. He was the pride of his commanding officer who told him at the end of his enlistment period that he would sponsor him for officer training school. Gordius, in a fit of trust (and ambivalence), told his mentor the truth about watching his younger brother and escorting his mother; as much as he was able, he took his father's place. Although this did not literally include sex, the tensions were there.

Mother was a survivor. Undaunted by unending labor and the deaths in her family, she kept on. A small dour woman, she compensated for her tenacity by avoiding any emotional commitments, particularly to her sons. The lack of affection, communication, consideration, and empathy were hallmarks of her stern care. She did have strong feelings about one thing: the need for her sons to stay with her always. The extended family was a culturally congruent concept and, as absolute matriarch, she counted on it. By encouraging guilt, inadequacy, and fear in her children she worked toward continuing this dependency, for to let them go would mean being alone in the world. Unfair. Gordius' best accomplishments were acknowledged, his worst highlighted. Girlfriends were vehemently discouraged. Mother was, excuse a term no longer in style, a schizophrenogenic parent.

Gordius had one ray of light in these dark days. He was picked up by an uncle for a monthly visit. The uncle was the only affectionate male in his life at that time. He attended to Gordius with enthusiasm. The love was frequent and literal. Gordius was sworn to secrecy. He knew that if his sex with uncle were discovered, his sole holiday would end. And, also, he cared much for this uncle.

Long after his younger brother had grown and left home, Gordius remained, not with satisfaction and not without attempts at his sexual orientation. But he had been celibate, he added. The CO said he'd have to think about that and dismissed Gordius. It was never clear whether she came with or without her husband's blessing, but that night the CO's wife visited Gordius to convert him to heterosexuality. Predictably, facing the very conflict he'd thought he'd left at home, he threw her out with editorial comment. The next day Gordius was sectioned out of the army on a medical discharge: homosexuality.

Back home with mother, he got a job on a delivery truck and tried to live harmoniously at home. The house rules from his side included absolute privacy for his room. Most important to him, mother was *never* to sit on his bed. Of course she did, and often. Gordius threw epithets, furniture, and generally caught his mother's attention.

She began taking him to the family physician for therapy. Her primary concerns were disobedience, tantrums, and homosexuality. The family physician was not a psychotherapist but undertook individual therapy anyway. He was the community medical expert. While Gordius was being seen, unknown to him, mother was allowed to watch and listen from an adjoining room. After her son's sessions ended she then consulted with the doctor to review the material. Gordius was 30.

Eventually Gordius saw through this procedure, refused to return to the unethical setting, and called the physician to tell him why. It was an important event for Gordius; he was able to confront this father-figure emphatically and effectively. He stood up to him and told him off.

The next day his physician died from heart failure.

While mother made full use of the event to consolidate her domination of Gordius, she had become ambivalent herself. She was becoming increasingly fearful, as was he, that his violence with furniture might eventually extend to her. Gordius was also, in his most recent feelings of guilt and failure, developing enough anger suppression and guilt to be suicidal. He wondered about his own sanity.

Given all of this, Gordius voluntarily committed himself, in rare cooperation with his mother, to the free public care of the state mental hospital.

INTAKE

All life is an experiment.

(Ralph Waldo Emerson, 1880)

The day always began early so at the end of the shift there would still be surf time. I was a post-doctoral clinical intern and this was my first intake session. Gordius was presented via paper as needing treatment for "homosexuality and disobedience," although the diagnostic description was "borderline schizophrenia."

Borderline in those days meant they didn't know what he was.

The Volunteer Services Coordinator, years ahead of her time, objected to homosexuality as a diagnostic category of mental illness. I supported her and added that unquestioning obedience to his mother as a psychiatric goal, particularly for a patient in his 30's, was not realistic. We were, of course, rewarded for this heresy by being assigned treatment responsibility for Gordius. Already responsible for 200 patients, I soon learned that any comment at intake was automatic commitment to taking on yet another individual case.

The Volunteer Services Coordinator, more seasoned than I, soon handed off her responsibility to the new volunteer art therapist. I began seeing Gordius for individual therapy once a week in my office.

GOALS

Perfection is finally attained, not when there is no longer anything to add, but when there is no longer anything to take away.

(Antoine de Saint-Exupery, 1940)

It was easy for Gordius to formulate his goals for success. Most important was to leave home, break away from mother. As to his sexuality, he didn't really want to abandon men; he just wanted to relate more positively to women. He was also fearful of his violence and wanted some control. For his suicidal feelings, he needed both better expression of his anger and a more satisfying vocational setting than the bread truck. Finally, he was afraid of becoming schizophrenic; he understood what his diagnostic label predicted, and he wanted some control of that as well. We agreed on all these goals.

MOTHER AND THE GOVERNOR

The greatest challenge for young people is to learn good manners in the absence of any example.

(Fred Astaire, 1981)

Shortly after therapy began, Gordius' mother called me to find out what he was saying about her. I explained that, because of his adult age, his confidentiality had to be protected. I referred her to a social worker for information in a general sense about the program. She did not take this easily, being particularly concerned about a comment from her son that the primary treatment goal was his freedom.

In another era this might have led to family or system work. But this was 1966 and mother chose a more direct route. She complained to the Governor of the state of Hawaii.

Hawaii is a small state with a big heart: her complaint was heard and considered. It took several months before she was finally told, "Dr. Morgan was correct in his approach." She called me one more time. "It's not fair," she said. "Why should *he* get the good therapist? *I'm* the one who worked so hard."

But mother didn't come in for treatment with another practitioner. In time she eventually talked her youngest son into returning home.

ART THERAPY

A portrait is a painting with something wrong with the mouth.

(John Sargent, 1920)

The volunteer art therapist, Mrs. W., was much loved by her patients. Not only were her classes fun but she taught them much about themselves. What wasn't true to begin with soon became so. For example, she explained at the outset that psychosis was communicated in art by greens and purples. While this had little empirical support in the literature, it soon became both a self-fulfilling prophecy and an important form of communication.

With Mrs. W., Gordius was confronted with a relentlessly positive female role model. In the beginning, he challenged her often. He painted her portraits in greens and purples. Unfazed, she had him copy cartoons of female faces and pointed out his turning straight line mouths into scowls. (Even male figures rarely were smiling; female ones never were).

He began to identify her favorites among his productions and say, "These are for Dr. Morgan." But it didn't work. She continued (and continues) to be his friend. One goal met.

At every one of our sessions he would choose some of his art to express feelings in individual therapy. In addition to speed sketching, copying, and other art therapy techniques, he continued to develop his own unique artistic style. A selection of these are included in this chapter.

TRANSFERENCE

The easiest kind of relationship for me is with ten thousand people. The hardest is with one.

(Joan Baez, 1989)

Gordius has a learned expectancy for a good father and a hostile mother. The art therapist had not fit well into the hostility mode and his original mother was not part of the hospital community. While I held the role of the father for a time, Gordius settled on a new target as "mother": the male psychiatrist in charge of our unit and my supervisor.

This is, of course, hindsight. At the time I had no insight into the increasingly hostile exchanges I was having with Dr. R. He had been gone my first months at the hospital during which time I had engineered a moratorium for his only treatment approach: ECT. He managed to take this in stride but it predisposed him to seek out alternate challenges to my work. There was no love between us and if I thought of him at all as a mother, it was only in the presence of two additional syllables. So, Gordius chose well. Dr. R. was clearly, even though the gender was wrong, a personality much like his own mother. Even the size and belief systems were the same. By violating small rules just before our sessions, he regularly triggered solitary confinement punishments from Dr. R. which voided our therapy. I objected, often seeing Gordius in his cell, and the battle was on. In time and with good supervision from my psychologist compadres, I finally saw what was taking place and made my peace . . . or at least worked with Gordius until he saw his role in maintaining the war and removed himself as cause of the battle.

This was a big breakthrough for Gordius. He began to realize his existential power: no longer was he a child unable to shape his life.

Concentrating now on his relationship with me, he began to make demands. Therapy twice a week: OK. Therapy daily: no. No? He warned me he could become violent if not given enough care. I asked him to visualize the violence. He did so: not against himself or others but a brick through an empty building's window. The answer was still no.

I called the ward and told him that he would be back but would break a window on the way. They thought I was a great prognosticator when the glass broke.

At our next meeting we went out and looked at the still-unrepaired window. "Still no extra sessions?" he asked. "Nope." The patient-therapist relationship had been clarified and limited. We both relaxed and got on with the therapy.

HOLIDAY

Whether one chooses celibacy or marriage, it will be repented.

(Socrates, 422 BC)

Gordius was making good progress in the hospital. He was getting along with others of both sexes, his art was flourishing and was much admired, and he had developed some control of his acts of violence.

By using visualization techniques, he was able to confront thoughts rather than hide from them and to express anger in his fantasies rather than his actions.

He also felt able to address his relationship with his mother. He got my permission, and hers, to spend a holiday weekend at home.

His brother away, it was a chance for Gordius to try to move his relationship with mother to a more positive level. First, though, he thought he'd stop by the order of Catholic brothers.

There he told them that he was successful in therapy and now wanted to begin a new life with them.

While Gordius had changed, they had not. Again he was evicted for calling them unchristian. They wanted no part of formerly gay priests even if celibate.

Gordius went home and, for once, opened up his sadness to his mother. He had neglected to realize that she, minus any therapy, hadn't changed any more than the brothers had. She sneered at him and told him he wasn't a man. As she said this she took the knife that had been carving their turkey and slammed it down next to him on the table. He grabbed the knife and growled. Mother fainted.

Holding the knife, he went through his exercises, in fantasy carving her up like the turkey. Suddenly he relaxed, realizing he need never harm anyone. With his thoughts free his actions were in control. He put down the knife.

Mother sat up with a sneer. He picked up the knife. Mother lay down again. He finally went over to mother, scratched her arm, and called the police. (This too was functional; she never invited him back that year.)

Sunday night. The police sergeant came to my house and asked me if Gordius was sane or crazy when he attacked his mother. A neophyte, I gave candor: I didn't know. This wouldn't do. The officer patiently explained that if crazy, he could leave Gordius at the hospital but if sane he had to book him. I also knew the medical director never wanted us to say patients were crazy in such circumstances for liability reasons (she had only the month before insisted on the sanity of a released patient that subsequently did homicidal sniping). I decided to interview Gordius.

Is your mother OK now? Yes. At the time you held the knife in your hand and she was beginning to sneer at you again, did you think of anything you could do besides scratch her with the knife? No. OK: you were crazy. The officer, relieved, left Gordius with the hospital. The medical director and I had a difficult meeting on Monday. But the therapy continued.

It was a turning point for Gordius. He never hurt anyone again, was master of his actions, developed more alternatives than the habitual self-defeating ones, and clearly left home for good. At least the home with mother.

LOVE AND SCHIZOPHRENIA

How complete is the delusion that beauty is goodness.

(Leo Tolstoy, 1901)

At ease with women, Gordius now developed a relationship with another male patient. He had worked through and abandoned the common fantasy that somehow his heterosexual married therapist would satisfy his non-therapeutic emotional needs and was now in love with a poetic compadre from his ward.

It went well until Gordius chose to paint his lover's disorder. Gordius painted his lover in green.

Since the lover also had Mrs. W. as an art therapist, he got the message and the relationship ended.

Now Gordius was concerned about his own sanity. If he could be fooled about a lover, couldn't he also be fooled about himself?

Much of my successful therapy had been based on the analytic (Bert Karon) and behavioral areas (Ray Denny, Stan Ratner) but the hospital supervising psychologists (Howard Gudeman, Robert Hunt) were very existential. Despite my resistances to learning, the power of these ideas coupled with the writings of Rollo May (later a friend of the family) took me to a new direction for this fear of Gordius. What I did in 1966 would later be popularized as "paradoxical intention." I labeled it: "seemed a good idea at the time."

I worked with Gordius on his existential progress in taking responsibility for his life. I told him he had the capacity, if he *chose*, to be schizophrenic. He also, therefore, had the capacity not to be. To demonstrate this I suggested he visualize what it would be like if he were schizophrenic. I was assured that his conception left no room for violence to himself or others. Rather it sounded much like the experience that early medical experimenters with LSD described. I then suggested he spend the next week being his version of schizophrenic. He agreed.

Much of the art from this period is in this chapter. He drew on his knowledge of schizophrenics in the hospital and on this artistic license. His hallucinations were more visual than auditory and his art was reflective in some cases of good schizophrenic art: trees with organs, the art therapy building with the inside on the outside. Occasionally he would be inconsistent and reality would sneak in: one picture had his first good self depiction at the time. This was actually quite congruent with reality, he was making a sane choice to travel through the experience of craziness. He had painted himself schizophrenic. He lost his fear of the borderline diagnosis and showed no further schizophrenic symptoms in the remainder of his year with me at the hospital.

DISCHARGE

Truth is stronger than fiction.

(*Experience*, Robert F. Morgan, 1990)

Gordius had developed some discharge plans. He had met his goals and was now committed to developing an outside career as an artist while living on welfare. Although what he planned was feasible, he was nevertheless terrified.

The only places he had ever succeeded in for long, away from mother, were the army and the hospital. The former was out of the question and the latter was about to be left behind. The hospital had become his home.

This was reflected in his art. A straw man walking up steps leading to nowhere was typical.

One day he left a drawing of a bird flying over a moat. I put it on the wall as always to wait for my consultant.

My consultant was a patient from a different ward who had moved through paranoid schizophrenia (he eventually got a Master's Degree in counseling at a state university) and visited me regularly to work on his discharge. In addition to library research, he was a first-rate interpreter of art from real experience. John Rosen had used ex-patients in therapy and I thought I might benefit from the same counsel.

My consultant didn't know Gordius but was always right about interpretations of his art on my office wall. Subsequent free association with Gordius invariably came to the same conclusion. Early on, my consultant had walked up to a sketch by Gordius of Christ on the cross faced by praying Mother Mary and a little brother (not quite the way the New Testament had it). I had merely interpreted it as more religious fixation and family enmeshment. My consultant put it more directly: "He's willing to be crucified if that's what it takes to get his mother and brother to bow down to him."

My consultant was also good at recognizing me in Gordius' drawings; that was also something I occasionally overlooked.

So on this day, only one month away from Gordius' discharge, my consultant walked over to the fleeing bird and said: "How long ago did the artist leave here?" "An hour." "Well, Doc, we still have time to catch him before he gets to the top of the Pali and dies of exposure."

Absolutely correct. Afraid of heaving through the front door, Gordius climbed the mountain of perpetual rain dwarfing the hospital. The rescue team brought him back intact. We kept working on discharge.

In the end I continued to see him on a monthly outpatient basis until I left the islands. He seemed happy and was generating some exceptionally fine art work. He continued his contact with Mrs. W. but we lost touch.

Ten years went by.

NO PLACE LIKE HOME

The only man who is really free is the one who can turn down an invitation to dinner without giving an excuse.

(Jules Rennard, 1899)

It was Christmas and I was visiting Hawaii's state hospital for the first time in a decade. We were seeing friends in the area and I thought I'd take an hour to stop by the place where I used to work. With the Hawaiian sense of personal history, the hospital still had my name in their literature as founder of the adolescent treatment program. I was enjoying seeing old friends and mixed memories. The hospital had shrunk from a census of 1000+ to a few hundred on wards for intensive or specialized care. The treatment had moved out to the community and a community college had taken over much of what used to be the hospital. My former supervisor and chief psychologist now ran the hospital, something that made me more optimistic than I expected to be about the institution's future.

Then nurse left from my era said, "One of the patients you worked with is here now. You remember Gordius, don't you?"

How sad, I thought. Had he visited once too often and been given ECT or other iatrogenic treatment (Morgan 1983)? Had he needed more therapy before he left?

"No, no," said the nurse, seeing my expression. "He's alright, it's just that Gordius is a street artist with very little money. Every Christmas he develops what we call 'seasonal schizophrenia'. He generates enough symptoms to join us for Christmas including our Christmas Dinner. He'll be well by New Year's Day. Gordius is an annual event here."

NOTE

Gordius' artwork follows.

REFERENCES

Morgan, R.F. editor (1983). *The Iatrogenic Handbook: A critical look at research and practice in the helping professions.* Toronto: IPI Publications Ltd. (Out of print: Available from author.)
Morgan, R.F. editor, (1985). *Electric Shock.* Toronto: IPI Publications Ltd.

Self-Image

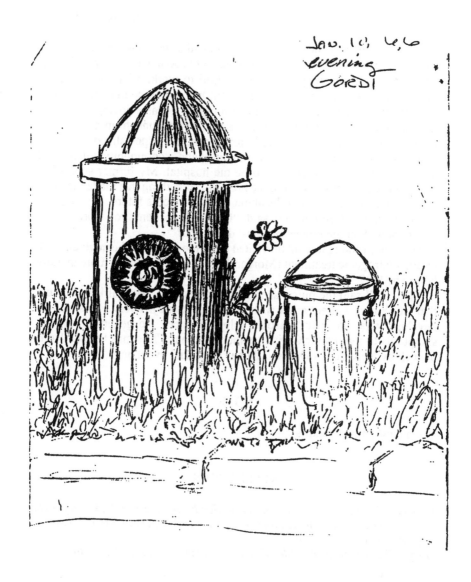

Self-Image

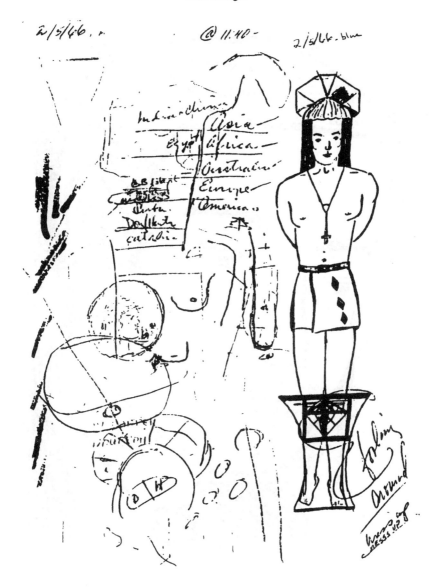

Psychotherapist

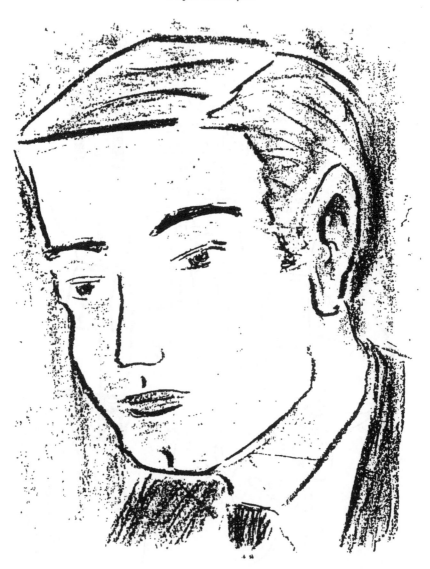

Art Therapist

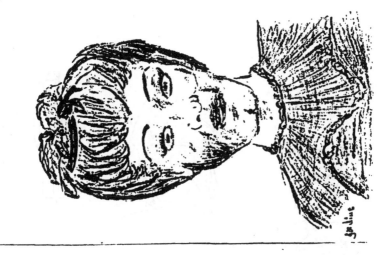

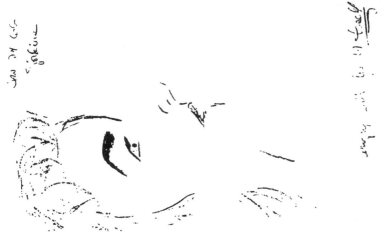

Art Therapy Technique: Frowning Women

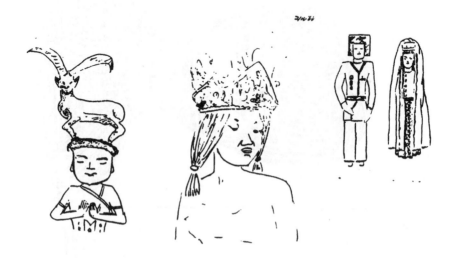

Art Therapy Technique: 2 Minute Family Portrait

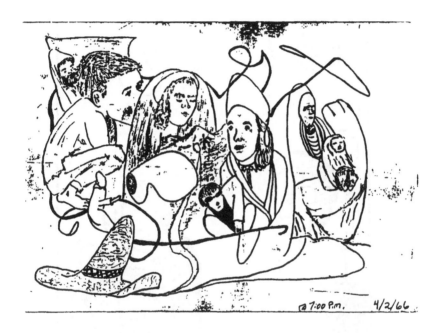

Another Family Portrait, Therapist Added

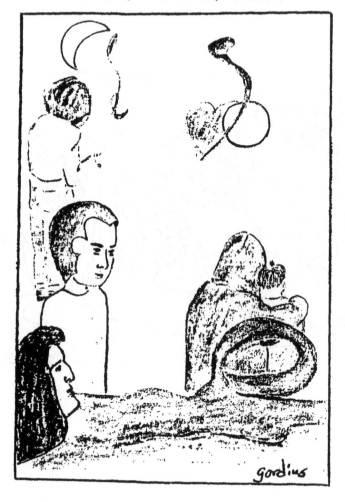

II.S.H HAWAII   APRIL 14, 1766

Distancing: Stained Glass Faceless

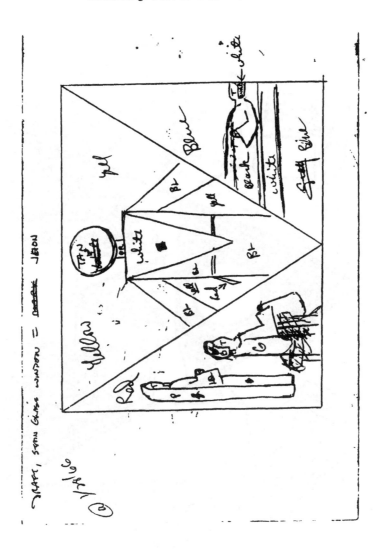

Distancing: Stained Glass Faceless

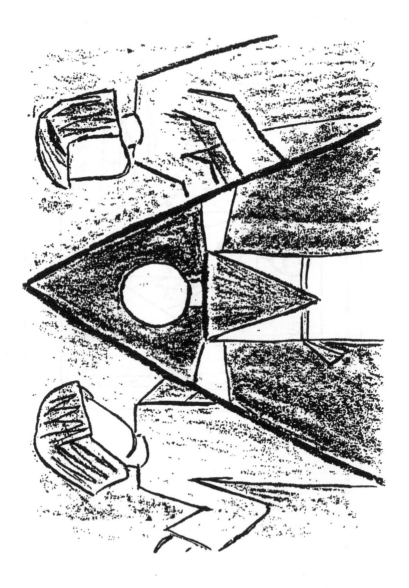

Distancing: Stained Glass Faceless

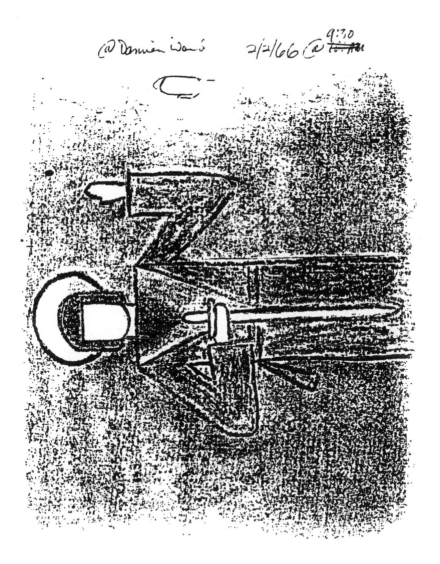

Family Portrait: Stained Glass With Faces

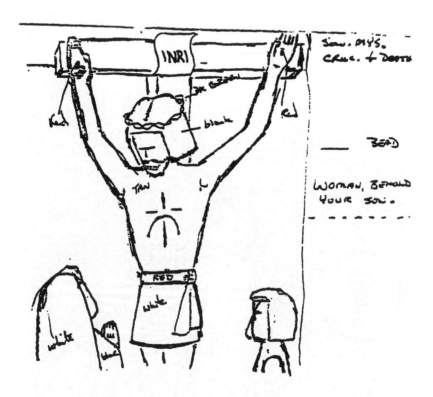

Family Portrait: Including Preceding Patient

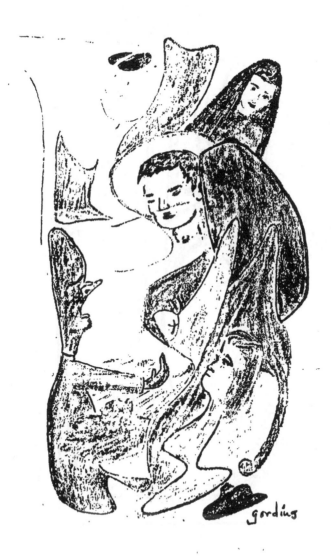

Family Portrait: (Original Monster In Green) "Life In Death"

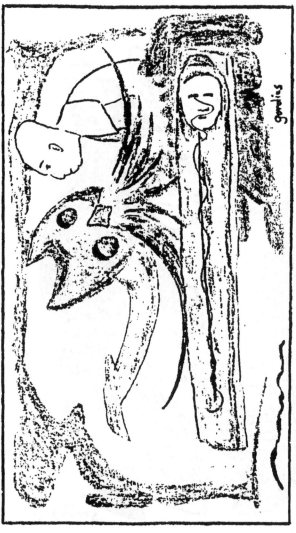

Parental Hierarchy: Gloomy Outlook For Sick Turtles

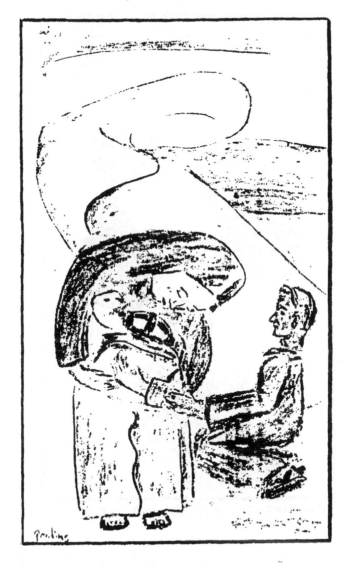

MAY 8 & 9, 1966 . H.S.H. _____

Vocational Exit

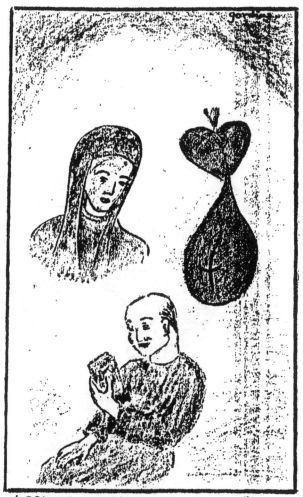

LOOKING AT "MY WAY OF LIFE."

APRIL 29, 66. H.S.H.

Vocational Problem

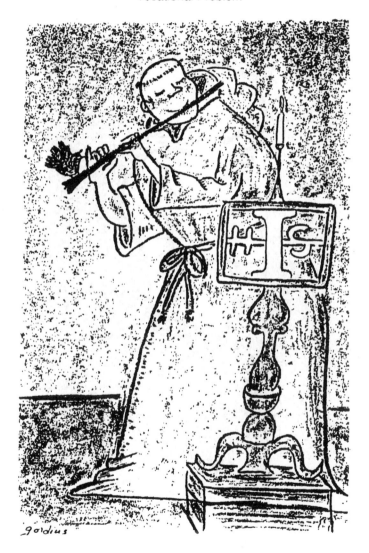

Artist's Insight: Portrait Of Poet And (Delusional) Lover

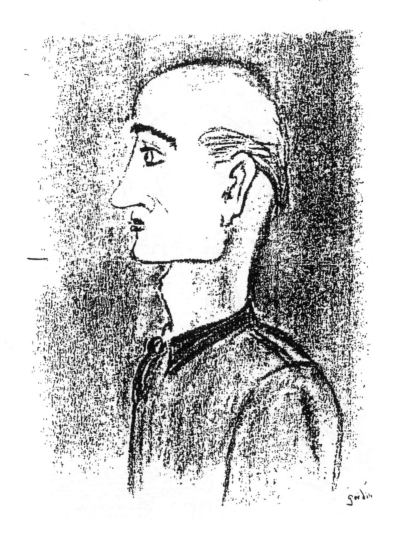

Paradoxical Intention: Schizophrenia Choice Art Morning Of Day 1

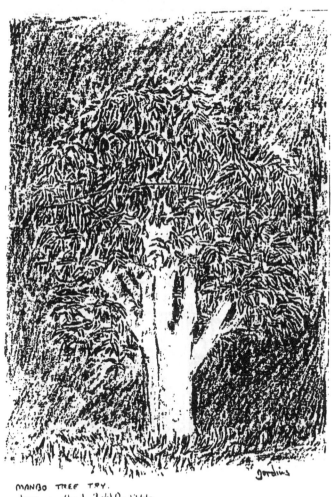

MANGO TREE TRY.
done on April 9+10, 1966

Paradoxical Intention: Schiz. Choice Art In PM: Art Therapy Building In/Out

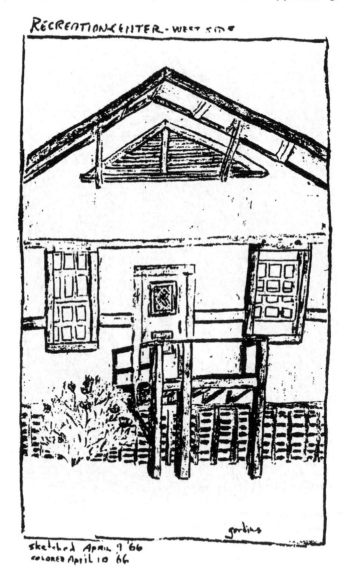

More On Schiz Choice Day: Afternoon Art And Tree Has Changed (Self Image +)

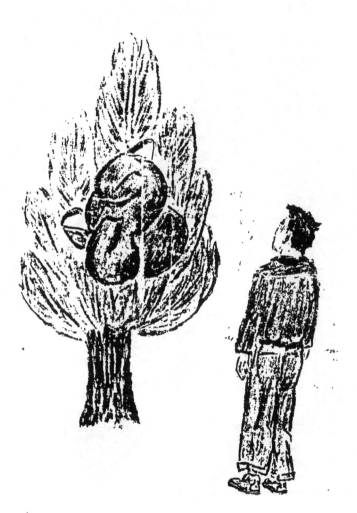

gordizs

Choosing Not To Be Schizophrenic But Still In Need

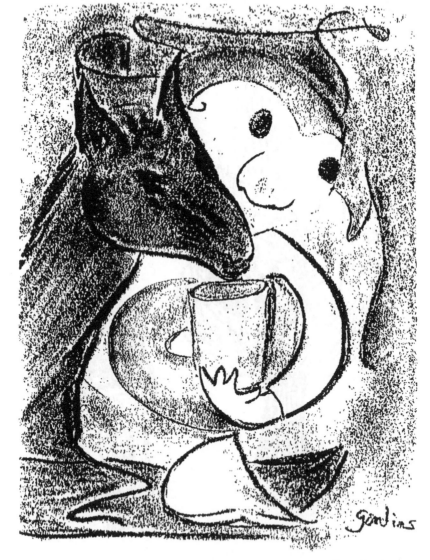

Stained Glass Curtain Call: Impending Therapeutic Interruption

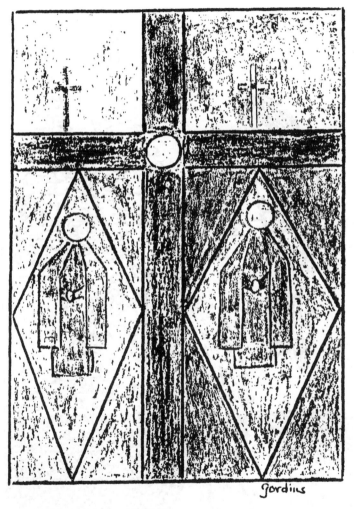

gordius

APRIL 28 1966. H.S.H

Health Anger At Therapist: Gone For A Week In A Good Cause

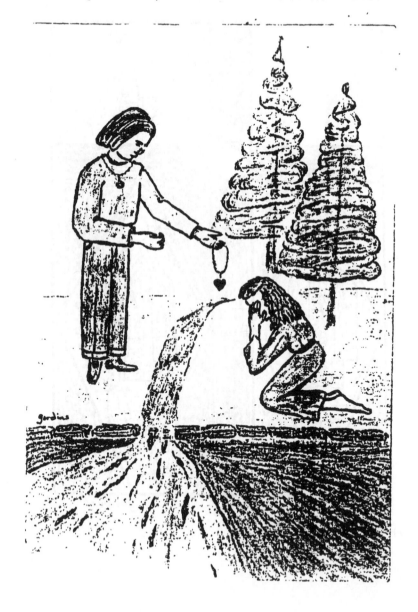

New Surreal Art Style Developing; Depression Saved For Therapy Hour

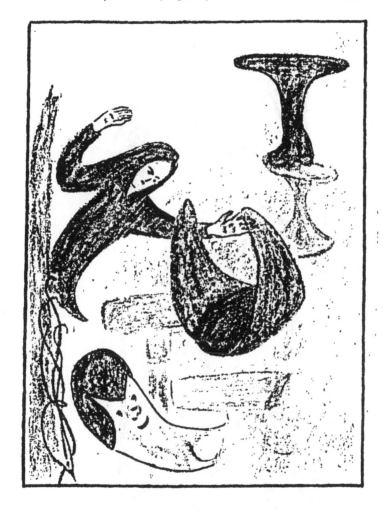

MAY 2 8 3. 196ä   11.ЗЛ.

More Surreal Style

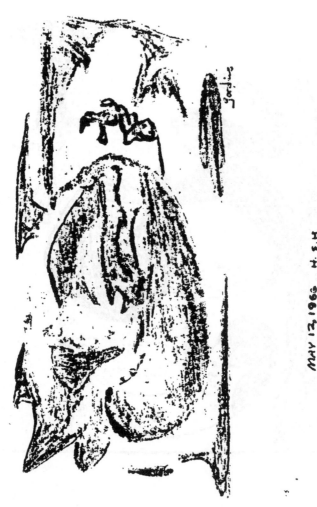

Flashback Curtain Call: Considering Discharge

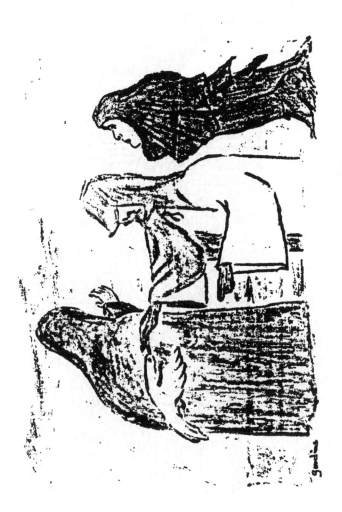

FEAST DAY OF ST. CATHERINE OF SIENA   APRIL 30, 1966. H.S.H.

One Flew Over: Run Away To Avoid Leaving

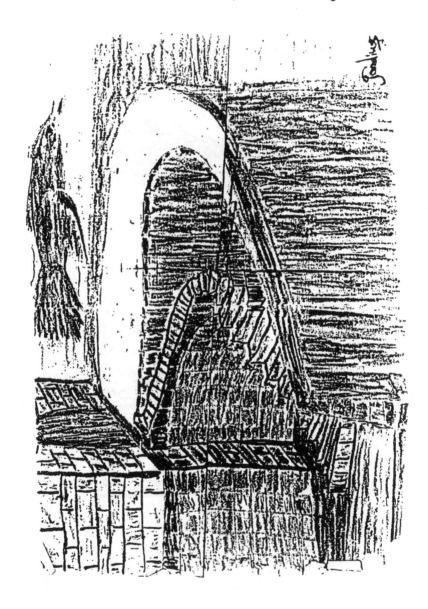

Therapist As Dragon: Discharge Approaching

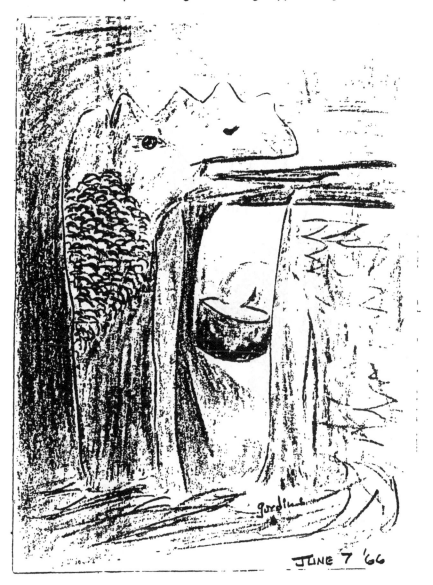

JUNE 7 '66

Straw Man and Stairway Leading Nowhere: Anxiety On New Life

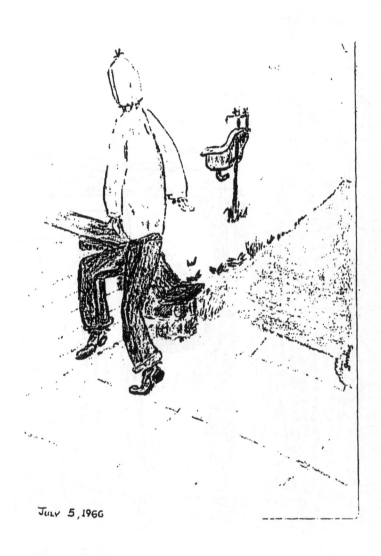

July 5, 1966

Ready To Leave: Art Style A And Accurate Self Image

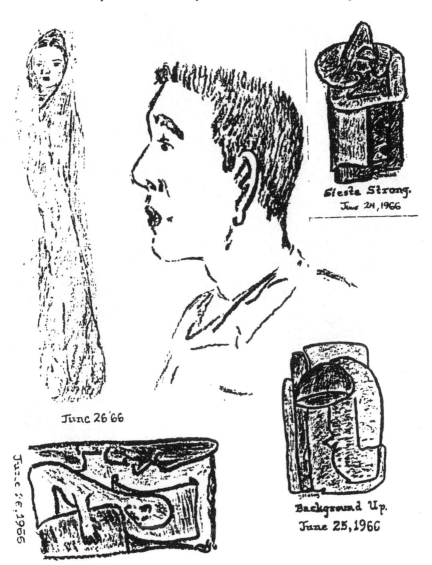

Siesta Strong.
June 24, 1966

June 26 '66

June 26, 1966

Background Up.
June 25, 1966

Art Style B: Discharge Week And Ready To Go

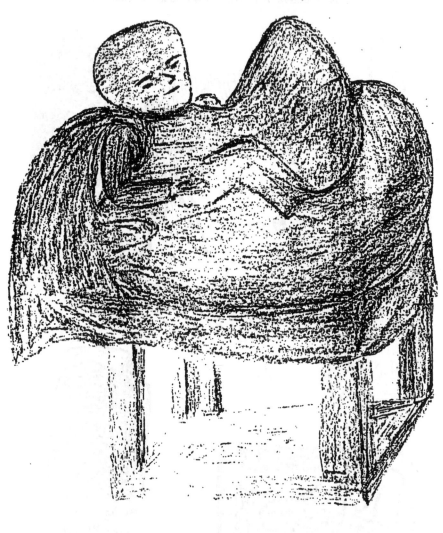

JUNE 20, 66

1990 Art Sample: Remembering Psychotherapy

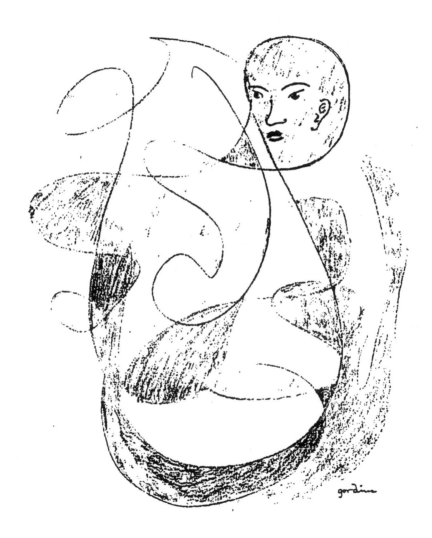

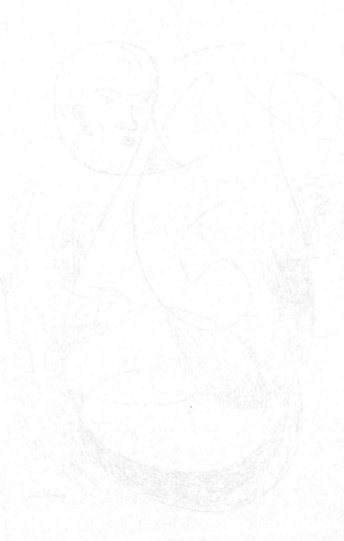

Working with the Families
of Schizophrenic Patients

Julian Leff
Ruth Berkowitz

SUMMARY. An investigation of working with families of schizophrenics in group settings as a means of assisting aiding in patients' expressed emotions and social contacts and in helping reduce relapse rates. *[Article copies available from The Haworth Document Delivery Service: 1-800-342-9678.]*

We have used the term "working with" in the title in preference to "therapy," because the latter implies that the family is the object of treatment and hence in need of it. This view characterised the therapy offered to families of schizophrenic patients in the 1950s and '60s, but was explicitly rejected by the new approaches that developed in the '70s and '80s. The earlier therapies were developed on the basis of the premise that the family was responsible for making one of its members schizophrenic. Consequently they were aimed at correcting the presumed distortion in the family, whether this was a problem with the parents' marriage (Lidz et al., 1957) or with communication between the members (Bateson et al., 1956).

We believe there was little or no evidence that such abnormalities occurred more frequently in the families of schizophrenic patients than in

Julian Leff, MD, is Professor in the MRC Social and Community Psychiatry Unit, Institute of Psychiatry, De Crespigny Park, London SE5 BAF.

Dr. Ruth Berkowitz is a Psychoanalytic Psychotherapist and Systematic Family Therapist. Mailing address: 18 Kensington Park Road, London W11 3BU.

[Haworth co-indexing entry note]: "Working with the Families of Schizophrenic Patients." Leff, Julian, and Ruth Berkowitz. Co-published simultaneously in *The Psychotherapy Patient* (The Haworth Press, Inc.) Vol. 9, No. 3/4, 1996, pp. 185-211; and: *Psychosocial Approaches to Deeply Disturbed Persons* (eds: Peter R. Breggin, and E. Mark Stern) The Haworth Press, Inc., 1996, pp. 185-211. Single or multiple copies of this article are available from The Haworth Document Delivery Service [1-800-342-9678, 9:00 a.m. - 5:00 p.m. (EST)].

families in which a member suffered from some other psychiatric condition (Hirsch & Leff, 1975). Nevertheless, these theories of family responsibility exerted a pervasive influence on psychiatric professionals and often led to families either being treated as grossly pathological or being shunned.

More recently, a new approach to family work began to emerge. The research background to this innovation was a series of studies conducted in the Medical Research Council Social Psychiatry Unit in London. These studies were focused on the emotional attitudes of relatives towards patients with schizophrenia. Measurement of the relatives' attitudes was achieved through use of a semi-structured interview, the Camberwell Family Interview (CFI), and a set of rating scales which became known collectively as Expressed Emotion (EE) (Brown and Rutter, 1966; Vaughn and Leff, 1976a). The ratings are made from audiotapes of the CFI and depend as much upon the rate, volume and tone of speech as on the content. The key ratings are of critical comments, hostility, overinvolvement, and warmth. In samples of relatives in western countries hostility always accompanies a high level of critical comments; however, in a study in north India, Hindi-speaking relatives expressed hostility at low levels of criticism (Wig et al., 1987). Each of the three negative components of EE is associated with relapse of schizophrenia over a nine month follow-up period after the patient's discharge from hospital. A high rating on warmth in the absence of high ratings on the negative components is associated with a lower relapse rate. These findings, which have been repeatedly replicated, suggested that relatives were capable of influencing the course of schizophrenia in a positive as well as a negative way. It is important to stress that in practice low EE relatives are not simply characterised by an absence of high EE attitudes. Far from being neutral or distanced from the patient, they have an extensive repertoire of coping skills. They are able to mobilise the inert patient without bullying, to defuse tension, to back off from conflict, and to create a supportive atmosphere without being overprotective. These are remarkable achievements when one considers that they have often developed in the absence of any professional input. Our experience of talking to low EE relatives raised the hope that if negative emotional attitudes could be modified, high EE relatives could be turned into an important asset for the patient's recovery.

Relatives are assigned to a high EE category if they score 6 or more critical comments during the CFI, express any degree of hostility, or score 3, 4, or 5 on the overinvolvement scale. Studies have now been conducted in a variety of cultures, and indicate that there is a wide range in the proportion of high EE relatives in the different settings (Table 1).

TABLE 1. Proportion of High EE households across cultures

Country	City	Group	%
Italy	Milan	Italian	70
UK	Salford	British	69
Poland	Cracow	Polish	69
US	Los Angeles	Anglo-American	67
Denmark	Aarhus	Danish	54
UK	London	British	52
US	Los Angeles	Mexican	41
India	Chandigarh	Urban	30
		Rural	8

There are two important implications of these findings. First, it is evident that in some cultures, particularly north India, only a minority of relatives show high EE attitudes, so that they cannot account for the first onset of the illness. Secondly, culture exerts a major influence on relatives' emotional attitudes to the schizophrenic patient. The nature of this influence remains speculative at present, but it appears that cultures which emphasize individual responsibility for success and failure, and which promote achievement through competition, also generate intolerance in relatives for the symptoms and disabilities of the schizophrenic patients.

There is other evidence against relatives' EE playing a causal role in the origin of schizophrenia, which derives from studies of non-schizophrenic conditions. Criticism has been found as frequently in the spouses of depressed neurotic patients as in the spouses of schizophrenic patients, and furthermore is associated with relapse of depression (Vaughn and Leff, 1976b; Hooley et al., 1984). High levels of criticism have also been recorded in the husbands of obese women (Fischmann-Havstad and Marston, 1984) and in the relatives of patients with Parkinson's disease (MacCarthy, personal communication), while overinvolvement and high criticism have been detected in the parents of anorexic patients (Szmuckler et al., 1985). These findings demonstrate that high EE attitudes can develop in relatives in response to a variety of psychiatric and physical disorders. The key factor is probably the relapsing or chronic course of the disorder rather than any specific constellation of symptoms.

Given these findings and the accumulating evidence from biological studies of structural and functional abnormalities in the brains of patients with schizophrenia, the assumptions underlying our intervention are that schizophrenia is primarily a brain disease and that some families with a schizophrenic member are functioning well on an emotional plane. These assumptions account for many of the differences between recent family interventions for schizophrenia and the earlier forms of family therapy used with this condition. These differences are presented in tabular form for ease of comparison (Table 2).

In running down the list, the first two differences have already been discussed, and are reflected in the aim of therapy. In recent interventions the aim is for the therapists to form an alliance with the family, enabling them to work together on the problems thrown up by living with a person with schizophrenia. The earlier interventions were often based on psycho-dynamic theories, and the therapists' insights were relayed to the family with the expectation of inducing change. In our experience of working with families of schizophrenic patients we have not found that they were

TABLE 2. Comparison between earlier and recent family interventions for schizophrenia

	Earlier interventions	Recent interventions
Disease concept of schizophrenia	A psychological response to family dysfunction.	A biological illness which can occur in well-functioning families
Role of family	Implicated in the aetiology of the illness.	Not a *causal* factor. Can influence *course* for better or worse.
Aim of therapy	To correct family dysfunction. The family is the client.	To help family cope better with the patient. Family is an ally in treating the schizophrenic patient.
Role of insight	Fed back to family to produce change.	Helps therapists understand family. *Not* fed back to family.
Role of therapists	"Traditional."	Within sessions: giving family information, advice and guidance. Outside sessions: linking family with services.

able to use the insights we provided. That does not mean that we reject the usefulness of family dynamics. On the contrary, we often utilise dynamic theories to understand the behaviour of family members to one another. Sometimes they illuminate the critical or overinvolved attitudes of relatives. We have also found the concept of countertransference helpful in understanding the ways in which power struggles in the family become echoed in the therapeutic team, and in tracing the origins of feelings of anger and helplessness in the therapists (Berkowitz and Leff, 1984). However we no longer make statements to the families based on psychodynamic insights.

The final difference in Table 2 concerns the therapists' role. In more traditional interventions therapists tended to reflect back clients' questions within sessions and not to undertake activities on their behalf outside sessions. In recent interventions therapists provide family members with factual information, answer their questions about the illness, medication, hospital practices, and so on, and give guidance. Outside the sessions they act as advocates on behalf of the families with the health and social services. There are often difficulties in persuading service providers to engage with the families of psychiatrically ill patients and with the patients themselves. This is particularly true of schizophrenia on account of the chronicity of the condition, and the diversity of services that is often required. The therapists are in a better position to facilitate engagement than family members by virtue of their professional status and their greater familiarity with the personnel and procedures involved. Sometimes a phone call to a colleague will achieve what the family has failed to accomplish in months of trying. On the other hand, it is important not to take over from the family the responsibility of continuing contact with appropriate services. Some relatives behave in a manner that alienates service providers, in particular being very critical of what is offered. It is more effective for therapists to work with the family on this attitudinal problem than to attempt to maintain links between disgruntled relatives and disaffected professionals.

STUDIES OF THE EFFECTIVENESS
OF FAMILY INTERVENTION

The recent family interventions have been evaluated in a number of controlled trials (Goldstein et al., 1978; Leff et al., 1982; 1985; 1989; 1990; Falloon et al. 1982; 1985; Hogarty et al. 1986; 1987; Tarrier et al. 1988; 1989). In all the trials patients have been maintained on anti-psychotic medication, often depot preparations, and have been randomly assigned to a family intervention or to individual treatment of one sort or another. However, our most recent trial was exceptional in comparing two forms of family intervention. As shown in Table 3, in our first trial (Leff et al., 1982; 1985) we adopted a similar design to the other studies, comparing a package of family interventions with routine care, in which the relatives received little or no attention. Our second trial (Leff et al., 1989; 1990) was aimed at teasing out the effective components of the package and involved a comparison of family sessions with a relatives group. It should be noted that this is the only study that included a family intervention aimed at the relatives alone.

The results of these studies have been remarkably consistent, showing a significant advantage for family over individual treatment during the first year of follow-up. In most cases this has been sustained during the second follow-up year, although the difference in relapse rates has been reduced, with the exception of Falloon's study.

In our most recent study, the two-year outcome was almost identical for patients in the family sessions and relatives group streams, even though they were not involved in the latter intervention. This shows that modification of the attitudes and behaviour of the relatives alone is sufficient to improve the outcome for the patient.

The two-year relapse rates indicate that these interventions are not preventing relapse altogether. Rather they are delaying it, over and above the postponement of relapse achieved by maintenance medication. In our own two trials, for those patients who relapsed during the two-year fol-

TABLE 3. Design of two consecutive trials of family intervention

All patients on maintenance antipsychotic medication

Trial 1 (Leff et al., 1982; 1985)		Trial 2 (Leff et al., 1989; 1990)	
Control	Experimental	Experimental 1	Experimental 2
Routine Care	Education + Family sessions + Relatives group	Education + Family sessions (patients included)	Education + Relatives group (patients excluded)

TABLE 4. Outcome of family intervention trials for schizophrenia

Relapse Rates (%)

Study	6-12 months		2 years	
	Control	Experimental	Control	Experimental
Goldstein et al. (1978)	48	0		
Falloon et al. (1982)	44	6	83	12
Leff et al. (1982)	50	8	75	33
Hogarty et al. (1986)	41	0	67	25
Tarrier et al. (1987)	53	12	59	33
Leff et al. (1989)		8*		33
		17+		36

* Family sessions
\+ Relatives group attenders

low-up, the average time from discharge to relapse was 9.2 months in the control group and 14.2 months in the experimental groups, an average delay of five months.

The convergent findings of the various studies might appear surprising when the terms used by the therapists for their interventions are compared; namely crisis oriented family therapy (Goldstein et al., 1978), behavioural family management (Falloon et al., 1982), psychoeducation (Hogarty et al., 1986), enactive and symbolic behavioural interventions (Tarrier et al., 1988). However, content analysis of the interventions employed reveals a considerable overlap between the various studies, with a common core of educational, problem-solving, and structural approaches (Leff, 1985; Strachan, 1986). Rather than attempting to present an overview of all the interventions, we will describe our own in some detail. Readers interested in accounts of the others should consult Falloon (1984) and Anderson et al. (1986).

In describing our programme we are aware of the need to specify in considerable detail the nature of our interventions, since some of our readers are likely to be unfamiliar with the involvement of family members in therapeutic work. For other readers with experience of this approach we crave indulgence for the basic level of our account.

FAMILY SESSIONS AND RELATIVES GROUPS

We have already noted that our intervention was given in two different contexts, family sessions in the home and a relatives group. The fact that patients were not included in the group dictated a different approach. Nevertheless many of the principles and the techniques were the same across the two settings. We will describe our intervention as applied in family sessions, and then outline the ways in which the group meetings differed. However, first it is necessary to explain the education programme, since it preceded both other modes of intervention.

THE EDUCATION PROGRAMME

The rationale for attempting to educate the relatives derives from the aim of moderating critical attitudes. A content analysis of critical comments revealed the surprising fact that only 30% were about the florid symptoms of schizophrenia, such as delusions and hallucinations. By far the majority of critical remarks were focused on the negative symptoms of schizophrenia: apathy, inertia, failure to participate in household activities, and lack of emotional response (Leff and Vaughn, 1985). Relatives generally viewed these behaviours as an integral part of the patient's personality rather than the manifestations of a disease. They considered that the patient was able to control them and consequently blamed him or her for laziness or selfishness. We thought that educating the relatives about schizophrenia, including the nature of negative symptoms, might change their perception of the patient's behaviour and lead to a lessening of criticism.

We wrote an education programme in language that was as simple and as free of technical terms as possible. It was divided into four sections, on the causes of schizophrenia, the symptoms, the prognosis, and the treatment and management. In the first section on aetiology we stated that there was no evidence that families caused the condition. We presented it as an illness which had a strong hereditary basis. In describing the symptoms we laid as much emphasis on the negative as on the positive symptoms, explaining that they were not under the patient's control, although they could respond to the right management. Concerning prognosis, we stated that some people with a first attack of schizophrenia recover completely and remain well for many years. The European concept of schizophrenia is broader than the DSM-IIIR category and enables one to make such a statement. We also cautioned that although most patients lose their delusions and hallucinations after drug treatment in hospital, they are often left with negative symptoms and require a long convalescent period to return to a more normal way of life. We emphasized the importance of maintenance drugs in the management of the condition, and the need for patients to avoid undue emotional stress.

At first we gave the programme in four sessions, but soon found that this was too strung out and condensed it into two. We held the education sessions in the patients' homes, usually while the patient was still in hospital receiving treatment for an acute episode of schizophrenia. We chose to visit the home because we thought that relatives would be more receptive on their own territory. We later came to realize that there were a number of other advantages in beginning the intervention in this way. We were always welcomed by the relatives, almost certainly because we had made the effort to reach out to them and because we were bringing them a gift they valued–information. Relatives often find it difficult to obtain from professionals the information they need to understand the illness and to manage it. Our decision to give the education programme in the home turned out to be a very good way of engaging relatives, an endeavour that has proved problematic for other groups offering intervention.

Because the education programme was self-contained, we were able to evaluate it separately from the other components of our intervention. We assessed its impact on the relatives by giving them a Knowledge Interview immediately before and after the programme. In the first intervention study we found that there were relatively few significant changes in knowledge and attitudes in response to education. Whereas before the education, 50% of relatives knew that the diagnosis was schizophrenia, after it all relatives knew the diagnosis. This is not a surprising finding, but it needs to be stated that some relatives were still unwilling to accept that the patient suffered from schizophrenia and continued to maintain their own view of the problem. Probably the most important effect of the education was a significant increase in optimism (Berkowitz et al., 1984). This indicates that learning factual information about the illness is less alarming than being left in ignorance to harbour fears and fantasies.

In the second study, there were other significant changes recorded. In particular, relatives were less likely to advocate negative coping strategies such as "he should pull himself together." There was also a decrease in the number of relatives who believed the patient could make himself worse. However, this important increase in tolerance occurred between the education programme and the nine month follow-up and is almost certainly attributable to the addition of the other interventions (Berkowitz et al., in press). In both studies, then, the education by itself made very little immediate impact. We were neither surprised nor dismayed by this, since we viewed the formal education programme as only the first step in familiarising the relatives with the factual information we wished them to acquire. We anticipated that education would continue throughout the period of contact with the families, and this proved to be the case. The same questions kept recurring, and it was only when the relatives were ready to receive and accept the information that they ceased. This will be a familiar experience to anyone practising psychotherapy.

As explained above, the education programme was given to the relatives while the patient was still in hospital, so the patient did not participate. The programme was written in the form of a small booklet, which has subsequently been published by the National Schizophrenia Fellowship. We always left the booklet with the relatives, to give them an opportunity to review the information as often as they wished. We also told them that it was up to them to decide whether to show it to the patient on his return home. In this way we evaded the decision ourselves as to whether the education should be given to the patient. We now feel more confident about sharing the information with the patient and trying to enlist them in understanding and managing the illness when possible. For instance, without explaining the nature of schizophrenia to the patient, it is difficult to provide a rationale for continuing with maintenance drugs once the symptoms have abated. The timing of education for the patient needs to be carefully chosen, ideally when the acute episode has subsided.

THE FAMILY SESSIONS

General Principles

However problematic the relatives' relationship with the patient may be, they are almost invariably willing to continue to provide 24 hour care for him or her. Consequently it is important for the therapists to acknowledge the dedication of family members and the burden of care that they shoulder. Therapists should avoid direct criticism of what family members do for the patient. It may be very difficult for the therapist to hold back criticism when s/he sees examples of poor coping behaviour. However, criticism usually has a negative influence either in making the relative feel more guilty or in mobilising their anger. This may be directed towards the therapist, leading to rejection of the help offered, or may be displaced onto the patient, increasing the high EE atmosphere. Therefore therapists need to be like low EE relatives themselves, avoiding criticism of the family, and instead encouraging change in a warm, supportive manner.

The time scale of this work is very long. Schizophrenia, even when episodic, is a life-long problem. Brief interventions are unlikely to be helpful to the families. Family sessions last one hour and are held once a fortnight for at least nine months, but sometimes continue for two to three years at a lesser frequency. The therapists need to persevere and to be content with very small changes over long periods of time. Furthermore, while relatives and patients are appreciative of the therapists' time and interest, they are unlikely to acknowledge the positive changes that have occurred imperceptibly. Therapists who attempt to convince the family that they have changed are more likely to provoke attempts to prove them wrong than to receive appreciation.

THE THERAPISTS SUPPORT GROUP

The need for therapists to avoid direct criticism of family members, to be patient for months or years, and to put up with little positive feedback impose a considerable emotional burden. For this reason it is necessary to establish a therapists support group. This comprises other therapists working with families of schizophrenic patients. In addition to its function in sustaining therapists over long periods of time, it allows them to let off emotional steam. All their negative feelings about family members can be safely ventilated in this forum. There is an additional emotional issue that the therapists group can deal with. We have observed that the intense emotions in high EE families readily become transmitted to the therapists without their being aware of the source. In particular, conflict within the family is often echoed by rifts within the therapeutic team, while feelings of impotence and hopelessness, which are commonly experienced by relatives, can be presented by therapists with respect to their work with the families (Berkowitz and Leff, 1984). The therapists group can help individual therapists to cope with these issues by identifying the source of the emotions within the family. This enables the therapists to plan ways of helping the family members to cope with them, rather than the therapists feeling defeated by a sense of hopelessness.

WHY TWO THERAPISTS?

We almost invariably expect two therapists to work together in the family sessions and in running the relatives groups. There are a number of reasons for this. Many families with a schizophrenic member are quite chaotic emotionally. There are numerous pressing problems to be dealt with, and emotions run high about each of them. It is like walking into the sea when there are strong undercurrents. It is easy for a therapist to lose control of the situation and to be swept this way and that by the conflicting emotional pressures. It is often the task of the second therapist to identify the danger, to stand steadily on the beach, out of reach of the undertow, and to throw the struggling therapist a line to effect a rescue. In practical terms this means taking over direction of the session for a while, and commenting on what seems to be happening, thus giving the other therapist time to recover his/her emotional balance.

Another advantage of two therapists is that it is easier to balance alliances with family members. Where there is a struggle for power and control in a family, it is natural for each family member to attempt to win one or both therapists over to their side. In order to work productively with the family it is necessary for therapists to make alliances with family members, including the patient. However these need to be balanced if the family is to achieve resolution of its conflicts. A single therapist can only ally with one family member at a time although he or she can shift alliances within a session. However the advantage of two therapists is that while one is making an alliance with a family member representing one side of a power struggle, the second therapist can support the protagonist on the other side, thus achieving a balance. It needs to be emphasized that these alliances are of course not permanent. Since the formation of alliances is often influenced by gender (the men against the women; a female relative attempting to attract a male therapist), it is useful for the therapist pair to be a man and a woman. However, there is not too much of a disadvantage in both being of the same sex.

A strategy that is available to two therapists but not to one is modelling conflict resolution. If the therapists disagree over an issue, they can bring the disagreement into the open and discuss it between themselves in front of the family in a calm and rational way to achieve a resolution. This may be a compromise, or one therapist may yield to the other, acknowledging that they are right. This provides a useful corrective to the family's heated response to conflict.

INTRODUCING THE INTERVENTION TO THE FAMILY

One of the questions that almost always arises in the first family session is, "why are you here?" This is an important challenge to the therapists. The family have not asked them to visit, so it is natural for members to question the purpose of their coming. Behind it is a concern about being considered "the patient," or anyhow in need of treatment. This is not surprising given the history of professional attitudes to relatives, which we have reviewed above. We have already emphasized that we do not view the relatives as "sick" or needing treatment, and the therapists' response must underline that stance. Our reply emphasizes the important role the family plays in keeping the patient well and is in the form, "we have come to help you help the patient." This statement incorporates a number of important assumptions which foreshadow the work to be done over the succeeding months or years. It is clearly stated that there is a sick person in the family who needs help. It is acknowledged that the family can take action which will help him/her. Nevertheless, it is suggested that they need the help of the therapists to augment their attempts to improve the patient's condition. We have found this kind of response to be entirely acceptable to relatives.

AVOIDING SOCIALISATION OF SESSIONS

For therapists to enter the family home is an unusual event, although there is a long tradition in the UK of home visits by the family doctor, and the development of community psychiatry has led to such visits by community psychiatric nurses and other psychiatric professionals. There is an inevitable ambiguity about the position and role of the therapists: should they be treated like guests or like staff in a service setting? How should they be addressed and how should they address family members? Should they accept offers of food and drink? The issue of the form of address is an important one since it involves matters of status and can reinforce or undermine hierarchies. The question of who wields authority in the family is often salient, particularly as the role of schizophrenic patient can confer power on the individual in subtle ways. Using a surname can help to reinforce intergenerational boundaries and bolster the authority of a parent. On the other hand, using a patient's full first name in preference to a diminutive form can stress adulthood and independence. It is sensible to begin by asking family members how they wish to be addressed. Formalities at the beginning of work with the family may be dispensed with later as they become increasingly engaged, and issues of power and authority are satisfactorily resolved.

We usually accept cups of tea or coffee and cake or biscuits when offered. It would indeed be churlish to refuse refreshments, when the family have often prepared them beforehand. This does not only represent politeness, but often is a way of showing gratitude for the visits. However, we do not interpret the gift, but accept it gratefully. Occasionally the relative's offer to make tea represents a way of escaping from the work of the session. If the therapists suspect this motive they should defer tea till later. Alternatively it can become the focus of useful work with an inactive patient. The relatives can be encouraged to persuade the patient to make the tea for the visitors. It must be recognized that sometimes families overstep the bounds and either lavish excessive hospitality on the therapists or attempt to engage them in social conversations, asking questions about their personal lives. This must be actively resisted or the therapists' ability to help the family will be undermined. It can be a difficult tightrope to walk, and therapists may find themselves arguing after the session about whether it was appropriate to accept the second slice of cake!

IMPROVING COMMUNICATION

Not all families with a schizophrenic member are poor at communicating. But in many high EE families the pressure of problems and of anxiety surrounding them leads to floods of speech which threaten to overwhelm the therapists. Furthermore in many such families the patient has withdrawn from conversation and is virtually silent. This can often result in family members talking as though the patient was absent, which in turn further reinforces the patient's withdrawal.

It is necessary for the therapists to establish some ground rules for communication. They sound very simple, but may take months to be observed and require frequent reminders to family members. First, only one person may speak at a time. In order to state this rule in a way that avoids the implication of criticism of family members, the therapists say apologetically that they can really only attend to one person at a time and as everybody has something important to say it is necessary to take turns. The second rule is that everyone is given an equal chance to speak. This ensures that the patient, and any other uncommunicative relatives, are not squeezed out of the conversation. The patient may be quite unused to having the floor, and when given a chance may remain silent. It is important for the therapists to prevent other family members from encroaching on the silence, and to reassure the patient that all present will sit quietly and listen in case there is something he/she wants to say. But if he/she prefers to remain silent that is quite all right. The value of this exercise is that it emphasizes the importance of listening attentively to others, even if they are saying very little. Relatives have often lost the skill of listening to others as they feel so dominated by their own concerns. It is frequently necessary for therapists to draw attention to something important that a family member has just said, asking others present if they heard it, and sometimes requesting them to repeat what they think the speaker said.

The third rule is that if a statement is made about a person in the room, they must be addressed directly. This ensures that patients are not talked about as he or she, as though they were not there. This practice just reinforces their sense of being a non-person, and furthermore some of them may already be plagued by third person auditory hallucinations. Another advantage of having to address someone as "you" is that it is more difficult to make really angry statements. It is much harder to say "you make a terrible mess everywhere" than "he makes a terrible mess everywhere." Thus insisting on direct communication tones down the negative emotion in critical remarks. Unless the therapists keep this rule firmly in mind, it is frighteningly easy for them also to slip into the habit of referring to the patient as he or she.

The successful establishment of these rules does more than improve the clarity of communication. It also begins to firm up the boundaries between individuals in the family, to redress the unequal distribution of power, and to reinstate the patient as a person, as deserving of respect as every other family member. Hence, although the rules appear simple, they are aimed at effecting substantial changes in the way family members relate to each other. That explains why it can take months before they are observed.

TEACHING PROBLEM-SOLVING

This involves a straight-forward behavioural approach, but is not that easy to implement for reasons we will discuss as we describe the successive steps. The first step is to explore the main concerns of the family. It is at this point that therapists often begin to feel overloaded by the number of problems that emerge, usually helter skelter. However, experience with families containing a schizophrenic member is useful in making therapists familiar with the common problems. These are often the manifestations of negative symptoms such as lying in bed till late, failing to attend to personal hygiene, and leaving their room in a mess. The problems tend to be phrased as complaints by the relatives about the patient, particularly when relatives score high on critical comments. The patient will generally need positive encouragement to present his or her view of what the problems are. Some patients, of course, deny the existence of any problems, which is one way of dealing with a barrage from the relatives.

The next step is to seek agreement between all family members on which problem is to be tackled first. This requires tactful negotiation by the therapists. Furthermore they have to be careful not to be diverted from their aim. Each problem raised by the family seems so pressing that they find it hard to concentrate on any one for long. As a result it often happens that just as the therapists believe they have achieved a consensus on a problem, a family member reverts to a previously raised problem and the whole family gets sidetracked into discussing it. It is necessary for the therapists to steer the family back to the agreed problem, gently but firmly. As the therapists may need to take this action regularly, it is best done with humour to avoid the family feeling criticised.

Once a particular problem is in focus, each person's response to it needs to be explored. If the problem is related to the negative symptoms of schizophrenia, as is often the case, high criticism relatives will tend to blame the patient. The therapists need to reiterate the information in the education programme that negative symptoms are part of the illness and that the patient is not being deliberately awkward. It is also useful to inform the family that these are common problems which occur in many families. This helps to reassure the family that they are not struggling with a uniquely awful situation, and suggests that ways of dealing with it may already have been worked out. It is essential that the patient's view of the problem be sought. This has the advantage of confirming the patient's experience, and also provides an opportunity for the therapists to establish the patient as an expert on schizophrenia. After all, nobody else in the family has inside information on the problem. This approach raises the status of the patient by turning his/her affliction into an asset, and begins to open up the relatives to an empathic understanding of the patient.

We have found that low EE relatives empathise with the patients without overidentifying with their experiences. By contrast high EE relatives reject patients' positive symptoms as rubbish or nonsense, for instance when patients report hearing voices they respond by saying they don't exist or are only imagination. Low EE relatives deal with this situation by acknowledging that the voices are a real experience for the patient but stating clearly that they do not hear them. High EE relatives are likely to be less critical of the patient if they gain a better understanding of the experiences the patient is going through. For this reason we encourage the patients to talk about their hallucinations and delusions in the family sessions. This also has the effect of demystifying the symptoms and reducing the relatives' fear of them. On occasion, after hearing the patient's account, a relative will reveal that he or she has experienced something similar at times, indicating the occurrence of minor untreated psychotic episodes. For example when a patient spoke about paranoid delusions, his sister recounted a time when she kept thinking there was a stranger hiding in the house. Revelations like this decrease the patient's feeling of alienation from other family members.

The patient's account of a problem can also contribute to the search for a solution. To take an example, difficulty in getting up in the morning is a common complaint, which often exasperates relatives. There are a number of different causes for this problem which the patient can help to sort out: excessive medication making the patient sleepy, a reversal of day-night rhythms so that the patient is awake and active into the early hours and asleep till the afternoon, a tactic to avoid social contact with relatives, or lack of any incentive to get up since there is nothing to do. Direct and precise questioning of the patient can help the therapists and the family to choose between these alternatives, and may also clarify the patient's understanding of the problem.

It is important to establish in considerable detail what each family member does when faced with the patient's problematic behaviour. Relatives are often reluctant to go into detail but this is necessary in order for the therapists to identify the ineffective coping behaviours which need to be altered. In addition to specifying what they do in these situations, family members need encouragement to verbalise what they feel about their attempts to cope.

Once each family member's perspective on the problem has been explored, the therapists need to break the problem down into small, manageable steps. To continue with the above example, if the difficulty in getting up in the morning is due to a reversal of day-night rhythms, the aim would be to help the patient go to sleep half-an-hour earlier and get up half-an-hour earlier. If the aim is set too high, the family is likely to fail and to become even more discouraged; whereas a small success will engender optimism. The family is asked to suggest ways of tackling the problem, in this case how to help the patient go to bed and get up earlier. The therapists need to be skilful in discriminating between high EE and low EE solutions and in steering the family towards the latter. A high EE solution would be to pull the patient out of bed in the morning (relatives have actually tried this) while a low EE solution might be to help the patient buy an alarm clock and set it, or to bring in a cup of tea at the agreed time.

After the family have reached agreement on a particular solution with the therapists' help, it is necessary to work out a detailed plan including what each family member will do, the precise timing, and the frequency of attempts. If the plan is too vague it is unlikely that it will be carried out. It is not essential that each family member is actively involved in the task, but it is important to stress that the whole family has the responsibility to see that it is attempted. This action reduces the burden on the patient, and lessens the likelihood of sabotage by one or other family member. It is often the case that at this stage someone will complain that "we have tried this before and it doesn't work." It is a mistake to rise to this challenge by promising good results this time, since this is unlikely to reassure a family used to failure. It is preferable to agree that it may not work, but to emphasize the value of persistence. Finally the therapists should let the family know that at the next session they will enquire about the outcome of the task. Whenever possible, each session should end with the setting of an agreed task and a reminder that the therapists will ask for feedback at the next visit.

If the family report that the task was successfully carried out, the therapists should be suitably encouraging, and must stress to the relatives the importance to the patient of appreciation expressed even for small advances. On the other hand, failure to complete or even to attempt the task must not draw criticism from the therapists. Having a schizophrenic member is already taken by the family as a sign of failure, and the therapists must avoid compounding this. Therefore they need to say that the task set was too difficult or that the timing was wrong. However, they do need to enquire into how far the family got with the task as this will help to identify the modifications required. A task such as the patient having to wash her underwear twice a week might have to be scaled down to once a week, while a task involving the parents going to the cinema together might have to be postponed until more work is done on their anxieties about leaving the patient alone.

REDUCING CRITICISM

We have already described some of the relevant techniques in preceding sections. The underlying negative attitude is ameliorated by helping the relative to separate psychologically from the patient, and to find sources of emotional satisfaction outside of the relationship with the patient. Lowering the relative's expectations for the patient (see below) contributes to this process, which often occupies a long period of time.

The situation facing the therapists depends to some extent on the patients' responses to critical relatives, which vary between social withdrawal and counter-criticism. Patients who respond to criticism with silence or by walking away do not provoke conflict, although they may exasperate the relative exceedingly. When patients are critical in turn, the mutual recriminations escalate and often lead to verbal abuse or physical violence. Another situation in families that commonly generates conflict is when one parent is critical and the other is overinvolved. The critical parent accuses their partner of being too soft, while the overinvolved parent sees the other as too harsh. Arguments frequently develop over the best way to handle the patient's problems.

Both these forms of conflict soon become evident in family sessions. The therapists have a fire-fighting role and have to extinguish conflict rapidly before it develops into a conflagration. This needs to be done firmly with authority, but without making family members feel criticised. When conflict arises the therapists should take control. They need to interrupt saying that both sides have good ideas about how to cope with the problem, but they both see it rather differently and it is necessary to discuss the different solutions and decide which one to try first. The aim is to promote a calm discussion of the alternatives instead of an emotionally fuelled argument which both are intent on winning. As noted above, the therapists may deliberately initiate a calm discussion of their own differences to model this approach to conflict resolution for the family.

When conflict arises between a relative and the patient, it also has to be halted, but this time with a comment by the therapist that it is evident how much the relative cares about the patient. Many readers will recognize this technique as reframing, that is, describing the interaction between family members in a way that emphasizes the positive aspects and plays down the negative ones.

It is evident that to halt conflict successfully, the therapists have to take a position of considerable authority and power over the family. This is necessary in the initial stages as these conflictual families are out of control emotionally, and are usually frightened by the outbursts of verbal and physical violence that regularly occur. Once the therapists have succeeded in controlling these, they can begin to hand back power and authority to the family members. This is essential in order for the family to learn to get on well together without the therapists.

In our studies, we have found that these techniques are generally effective in reducing criticism by the nine month follow-up.

REDUCING OVERINVOLVEMENT

Overinvolvement is more difficult to alter than criticism and requires a longer time-scale of intervention. We have observed small reductions in overinvolvement over nine months, but significant changes take two years or more to effect. This is probably because overinvolvement is of much longer standing than criticism, often dating from the patient's early childhood. It is ineffective to concentrate on the overinvolved parent alone, since both partners contribute to the bond. Work with both is required to achieve some degree of emotional separation.

It is not difficult for both partners to appreciate the importance of increasing the patient's independence. Indeed many parents are only too aware of what has become known as the When I Am Gone syndrome; the foreboding that no one will be available to take over their role in caring for the patient after their death. But even so it is hard for both partners to begin to let go of one another. The relative needs reassurance that nothing terrible will happen to the patient if s/he begins to relax their vigilance. At first even leaving the patient alone at home for half-an-hour may provoke extreme anxiety. It is necessary for the therapists to bring into the open the fears the relative harbours about what awful events might occur in their absence. It is often a great relief for the relative to be given permission by the therapists to lay down the burden of care for a brief period. We formulate this permission in terms of the relative having spent so much time and energy in caring for the patient that they have earned some respite.

Work with the patient is focused on building up their confidence that they can cope on their own, at least for a brief spell to start with. Once the first step has been taken, the work becomes a little easier, since the relative experiences a sense of relief at giving up some of the responsibility, and the patient a sense of achievement in coping by her/himself. However, the tug to return to a state of mutual inter-dependence, which is both uncomfortable and comfortable, remains strong, and progress is often slow and incremental. A healthy sibling in the family is a potential ally, to be made use of for accompanying the patient in excursions out of the home. They can also introduce the patient to a peer group with whom to socialise. However, a sibling may feel too embarrassed to establish contact between their friends and the patient. Furthermore mutual envy may develop; the patient being envious of the sibling's educational, occupational and social achievements, while the sibling envies the special position the patient occupies in the affections of the overinvolved parent. This may prove an insurmountable barrier to co-operation.

A useful technique in preparing the ground for separation is to ask the parent to recount how s/he left the parental home. This reminds the parent that independence from parents is a natural thing to aim at, and also rehearses the emotions that parent and patient will experience in the process. It is worth emphasizing here that the emotions aroused need to be worked through before any meaningful separation can be achieved. Attempts to part patient and relative forcibly, for example by moving the patient into sheltered accommodation, without this preparatory work will almost certainly end in failure. In only a minority of families we have worked with has the patient eventually moved out. But in the majority of overinvolved relationships patient and relative have managed to establish independent life styles, albeit under the same roof.

EXPANDING SOCIAL NETWORKS

Families with a schizophrenic member start off with average sized social networks, but with the passage of time the networks tend to shrink. This is a consequence of the family's embarrassment at taking the patient to social gatherings of friends and relatives and of inviting visitors to their home, as well as social withdrawal by the patient. It is not uncommon to find a middle-aged schizophrenic patient being cared for by an elderly mother, neither having any social life outside of the home. The burden of care is much more difficult to sustain in the absence of social support, and moreover the patient and relatives are forced into each other's company.

The therapists' aims are to encourage relatives to re-establish social contacts with friends and relatives, and to link up the patient with people of their own age. Relatives are often quite reluctant to make the necessary changes in social activity, partly because of the issue of separation from the patient which we have discussed above. It is worth noting that the therapists' act of joining the family itself expands their social network and acts as a stepping stone to further contacts. The same is true of the relatives group, which we will give an account of later.

With respect to the patient, deficient social skills may prove a major obstacle to establishing friendships outside the family. Patients often find it less threatening to attend a club frequented by other psychiatrically ill people than to mix with healthy individuals. Although falling short of the ideal, this is preferable to social isolation. As with the relative, the first step in making social contact is usually the most difficult for the patient. The therapists need to arrange for a community worker to accompany the patient on the first visit to a club or drop-in centre, or failing this for one of the therapists to go with the patient. If successful, this approach has the effect of reducing social contact between patient and relatives, which is one of the major aims of our interventions.

REDUCING SOCIAL CONTACT

We have explained above that the earlier naturalistic studies identified low social contact between patient and relative as a moderating influence on the effect of high EE attitudes. Patients who are able to distance themselves from relatives at moments of tension are less vulnerable to relapse. Some patients appear to use social withdrawal as a protective strategy, while some low EE relatives encourage it themselves, for instance one mother would suggest to her son that he take the dog out for a walk when the situation between them became tense. High EE relatives usually find it difficult to disengage themselves or the patient from tense encounters, so that therapists need to explain the value of "time out" for the patient and cooling off for the relative. The distancing can begin in a very concrete way in the family sessions. Therapists are required to note the seating arrangements in each session. Overinvolved relatives often take a seat next to the patient. At some stage, but not in the first encounter with the family, a therapist may suggest that s/he changes places with the patient. This therapist will then support the overinvolved relative in the "absence" of the patient, while the other therapist will support the patient's more separate position. It is surprising what a difference this strategy can make to the structure of family interaction.

We have already dwelt on ways of increasing leisure activities for patients and relatives. We also need to consider occupation. The patient is often unemployed, and the relatives may have retired or even have given up work to look after the patient. In the latter case, the therapists persistently encourage the relative to resume work again. If the relative has retired, work is done on finding an interest that the relative is likely to enjoy and persuading him or her to attend classes during the day or evening. These are available very cheaply in the UK as part of adult education. To cater to the patient's needs, a place is sought in some form of sheltered occupation. In the UK placements are available in day hospitals, day centres and sheltered workshops. There are often waiting lists for such facilities, and this is one example of a situation in which the therapists can usefully act as intermediaries between the family and the service providers.

LOWERING EXPECTATIONS

It is quite usual to find that relatives expect the patient to be completely cured on discharge from hospital, particularly if it is the first episode of illness. We have explained above our emphasis on the negative symptoms and their persistence for long periods of time. The therapists repeatedly stress the value of very small advances by the patient, and discourage relatives from putting pressure on the patient to return immediately to full-time work or education. This is a particular problem with middle class parents, who generally have high aspirations for their children and may not wish to consider more realistic alternatives. When a family is caring for a more disabled patient, it should be explained that, rather than expecting positive changes, preventing deterioration is a considerable achievement.

It is common for relatives to experience a deep sense of loss of the person they knew intimately before the illness developed. This can be particularly painful when the patient affords occasional glimpses of their familiar self, keeping hope alive that they will one day recover their undamaged personality. Relatives need to be given the opportunity to grieve over the lost and valued person and to come to terms with the reality of an individual whose ability to respond emotionally may be quite restricted. It is upsetting for the patient to share the relative's grief, which is best dealt with either in sessions with the relative alone or in the relatives group.

THE RELATIVES GROUP

The reader will have realized that there is no overarching theory that informs our work with families, although we have clearly defined aims derived from a substantial body of previous research. We are prepared to use any technique that helps us achieve these aims, and have borrowed from a number of different schools. This eclectic approach applies as much to the relatives group as to family sessions, but there are some advantages and some disadvantages of the former compared with the latter, which we will now explore. The following description is brief for reasons of space. The interested reader will find a fuller account in Berkowitz et al. (1981).

A major advantage of the group is that it can be constituted of both high EE and low EE relatives. When ways of tackling a particular problem are asked for, low EE relatives are likely to suggest helpful methods of coping which the therapists can then endorse. Relatives find it easier to accept suggestions from each other than from the therapists. They can always disqualify what the therapists say on the grounds that they have had no experience of living with a schizophrenic patient. Obviously they cannot reject the suggestions of other relatives for that reason. Furthermore relatives can be much more blunt with each other than therapists would dare to be. They appear capable of taking more forceful statements from other relatives in the group than they could from the therapists.

Because patients are not present in the group, the therapists can allow relatives more latitude in letting off steam than they would in family sessions. Anger, grief and guilt can be dealt with more openly in the group than in the home, where the patient needs to be protected against such intense emotions expressed by the relatives. However, the therapists have to exert some control in the group to prevent one relative dominating a session with his/her emotional needs. As in the family sessions, therapists try to give each relative present an equal share of the time. However when a new relative joins the group, they are encouraged to tell their story. All other members present are asked to give a brief version of their circumstances. This helps the new member to control the detail of their contribution, and to compare their situation with others. This recounting provides a useful, non-threatening way of enabling a new member to join the group. Not all relatives are comfortable hearing the experiences of other families. Relatives of patients with a first episode of schizophrenia in particular may be dismayed to hear of patients with long histories of frequent relapses and hospitalisations. Sometimes such relatives refuse to return to the group. On the other hand many relatives benefit from others' histories. They may feel relieved that they are not so badly off by comparison with others, they may be heartened by the ability of families to survive years of travail, or may even gain from seeing themselves mirrored in others without necessarily acknowledging it.

The group is open-ended so that relatives come and go as they see fit. It is held once a fortnight for an hour and a half, and on average each relative attends once a month. There are no interventions based on the group process.

We have referred above to the need to expand relatives' social networks. The group automatically fulfils this function, and relatives often form friendships with other group members and meet them socially outside the formal sessions.

The main disadvantage of the group is that the therapists cannot directly observe interactions between relatives and patients, which can be very informative. Therefore it is often appropriate to combine the group with family sessions held in parallel.

CONCLUSIONS

Our research has shown that if relatives attend a group, the reductions in EE, social contact and the patients' relapse rate are very similar to those achieved by family sessions. However, if the group is offered on its own, nearly half the families fail to engage. The group is obviously less expensive in terms of time and personnel than family sessions, since two therapists can work with six to eight families with one fortnightly meeting. In our first trial we used a combination of the two modes of working with families and found that almost all relatives attended the group. Therefore this is what we now recommend, namely two or three preliminary family sessions during which the relatives are invited to join the group. An occasional family session may still be required from time to time, but the majority of families will respond well to this approach. However there will always be some relatives who are unable or unwilling to attend a group. The reasons may be valid, for instance inability to take time off work, severe agoraphobia, or a physical illness, or may be a way of avoiding exposure to other relatives. Either way, therapists need to retain the flexibility to hold sessions in the home, since in the families who will not attend groups and who thus receive no professional help the patients have the worst outcome of all.

REFERENCES

Anderson, C. M., Reiss, D. J. and Hogarty, G. E. (1986) *Schizophrenia in the Family: A Practitioner's Guide to Psychoeducation and Management*. New York: Guilford Press.

Bateson, G., Jackson, D. D., Haley, J. and Weakland, J. H. (1956) Toward a theory of schizophrenia. *Behaviour Science, 1*, 251-264.

Berkowitz, R., Kuipers, L., Eberlein-Vries, R. and Leff, J. (1981) Lowering expressed emotion in relatives of schizophrenics. In (ed. M.J. Godstein) *New Developments in Interventions with Families of Schizophrenics*. London: Jossey-Bass.

Berkowitz, R. and Leff, J. (1984) Clinical teams reflect family dysfunction. *Journal of Family Therapy, 6*, 211-233.

Berkowitz, R., Shavit, N. and Leff, J. (in press) Educating relatives of schizophrenic patients. *Social Psychiatry and Psychiatric Epidemiology*.

Brown, G.W. and Rutter, M. (1966) The measurement of family activities and relationships: a methodological study. *Human Relations, 19*, 241-263.

Falloon, I.R.H. (1984) *Family Management of Mental Illness: A Study of Clinical, Social and Family Benefits*. Baltimore: Johns Hopkins University Press.

Falloon, I. R. H., Boyd, J. L., McGill, C.W., Razani, J., Moss, H. B. and Gilderman, A. M. (1982) Family management in the prevention of exacerbations of schizophrenia. *New England Journal of Medicine, 306*, 1437-1440.

Falloon, I. R. H., Williamson, M., Razani, J., Moss, H. B., Gilderman, A. M. and Simpson, G. M. (1985) Family versus individual management in the prevention of morbidity of schizophrenia: I. Clinical outcome of a two-year controlled study. *Archives of General Psychiatry, 42*, 887-896.

Fischmann-Havstad, L. and Marston, A. R. (1984) Weight loss maintenance as an aspect of family emotion and process. *British Journal of Clinical Psychology, 23*, 265-271.

Goldstein, M. J., Rodnick, E. H., Evans, J. R., May, P. R. A. and Steinberg, M. R. (1978) Drug and family therapy in the aftercare treatment of acute schizophrenia. *Archives of General Psychiatry, 35*, 169-177.

Hogarty, G. E., Anderson, C. M., Reiss, D. J., Kornblith, S. J., Greenwald, D. P.,

Javna, C. D. and Kadonia, M. J. (1986) Family psychoeducation, social skills training, and maintenance chemotherapy in the aftercare treatment of schizophrenia: I. One-year effects of a controlled study on relapse and Expressed Emotion. *Archives of General Psychiatry, 43*, 633-642.

Hogarty, G. E., Anderson, C. M. and Reiss, D. J. (1987) Family psychoeducation, social skills training and medication in schizophrenia: The long and the short of it. *Psychopharmacology Bulletin, 23*, 12-13.

Hooley, J. M., Orley, J. and Teasdale, J. D. (1986) Levels of Expressed Emotion and relapse in depressed patients. *British Journal of Psychiatry, 148*, 642-647.

Leff, J. P. (1985) Social factors and maintenance neuroleptics in schizophrenic relapse: An integrative model. *Integrative Psychiatry, 3*, 72-88.

Leff, J. P., Kuipers, L., Berkowitz, R., Eberlein-Fries, R. and Sturgeon, D. (1982) A controlled trial of social intervention in schizophrenic families. *British Journal of Psychiatry, 141*, 121-134.

Leff, J. P., Kuipers, L., Berkowitz, R. and Sturgeon, D. (1985) A controlled trial of social intervention in the families of schizophrenic patients: two-year follow-up. *British Journal of Psychiatry, 146*, 594-600.

Leff, J. P., Berkowitz, R., Shavit, N., Strachan, A., Glass, I. and Vaughn, C. (1989) A trial of family therapy vs a relatives' group for schizophrenia. *British Journal of Psychiatry, 154*, 58-66.

Leff, J. P., Berkowitz, R., Shavit, N., Strachan, A., Glass, I. and Vaughn, C. (1990) A trial of family therapy vs a relatives' group for schizophrenia: A two-year follow-up. *British Journal of Psychiatry, 157*, 571-577.

Leff, J. P. and Vaughn, C. (1985) *Expressed Emotion in Families: Its Significance for Mental Illness.* New York: Guilford.

Lidz, T., Cornelison, A. R., Fleck, S. and Terry, D. (1957) The intrafamilial environment of the schizophrenic patient. I. *Psychiatry, 20*, 329-342.

Strachan, A. M., Leff, J. P., Goldstein, M. J., Doane, J. and Burtt, C. (1986) Emotional attitudes and direct communication in the families of schizophrenics: A cross-national replication. *British Journal of Psychiatry, 149*, 279-287.

Szmuckler, G. I., Berkowitz, R., Eisler, I., Leff, J. and Dare, C. (1987) Expressed Emotion in individual and family settings: a comparative study. *British Journal of Psychiatry, 151*, 174-178.

Tarrier, N., Barrowclough, C., Vaughn, C., Bamrah, J. S., Porceddu, K., Watts, S. and Freeman, H. (1988). The community management of schizophrenia: a controlled trial of a behavioural intervention with families to reduce relapse. *British Journal of Psychiatry, 153*, 532-542.

Tarrier, N., Barrowclough, C., Vaughn, C., Bamrah, J.S., Porceddu, K., Watts, S. and Freeman, H. (1989) Community management of schizophrenia: a two-year follow-up of a behavioural intervention with families. *British Journal of Psychiatry, 154*, 625-628.

Vaughn, C. E. and Leff, J. P. (1976a) The measurement of expressed emotion in the families of psychiatric patients. *British Journal of Clinical and Social Psychology, 15*, 157-165.

Vaughn, C. E. and Leff, J. P. (1976b) The influence of family and social factors on the course of psychiatric illness: a comparison of schizophrenic and depressed neurotic patients. *British Journal of Psychiatry, 129,* 125-137.

Wig, N. N., Menon, D. K., Bedi, H., Leff, J., Kuipers, L., Ghosh, A., Day, R., Korten, A., Ernberg, G., Sartorius, N. and Jablensky, A. (1987) Expressed emotion and schizophrenia in North India. II. Distribution of expressed emotion components among relatives of schizophrenic patients in Aarhus and Chandigarh. *British Journal of Psychiatry, 151,* 160-165.

WHO Studies on Schizophrenia:
An Overview of the Results
and Their Implications
for the Understanding of the Disorder

Giovanni de Girolamo

SUMMARY. In this paper we shall briefly describe the three main studies carried out by World Health Organization on schizophrenia, namely:

1. the International Pilot Study of Schizophrenia (IPSS);
2. the study on impairments and disabilities in schizophrenic patients;
3. the study on determinants of outcome of severe mental disorders.

We shall then discuss the main results of these studies and their implications for a general understanding of this disorder.

Giovanni de Girolamo is affiliated with the Division of Mental Health, World Health Organization, 1211 Geneva 27 (CH).

This paper is based on the data and experience obtained during the WHO Projects on 'the International Pilot Study of Schizophrenia,' on the 'Study on impairments and disabilities in schizophrenia patients,' and on 'The determinants of the outcome of severe mental disorders,' projects sponsored by the World Health Organization, and funded by the World Health Organization, the National Institute of Mental Health (USA) and the participating field research centres. A full list of all investigators and staff involved in these projects is presented in the official published reports of the studies.

The opinions expressed in this paper are solely responsibility of the author and do not reflect the views of the World Health Organization.

[Haworth co-indexing entry note]: "WHO Studies on Schizophrenia." de Girolamo, Giovanni. Co-published simultaneously in *The Psychotherapy Patient* (The Haworth Press, Inc.) Vol. 9, No. 3/4, 1996, pp. 213-231; and: *Psychosocial Approaches to Deeply Disturbed Persons* (eds: Peter R. Breggin, and E. Mark Stern) The Haworth Press, Inc., 1996, pp. 213-231. Single or multiple copies of this article are available from The Haworth Document Delivery Service [1-800-342-9678, 9:00 a.m. - 5:00 p.m. (EST)].

213

INTRODUCTION

Some twenty million people in the world suffer from schizophrenia. The disease usually starts early and often has a chronic, disabling course. The overall cost of the disorder, both direct and indirect, is huge. The burden caused to the patient's family is very heavy and both patients and their relatives often experience disadvantages because of the stigma associated with the disorder, sometimes over generations. Schizophrenia is a major public health problem. These facts were among the reasons which have made the World Health Organization pay special attention to the problem of schizophrenia and launch or stimulate studies aimed at a better understanding of schizophrenia and at finding ways to deal with it. The programme of collaborative clinical and epidemiological research on schizophrenia, which started in the late 1960s, also aimed to develop a reliable methodology for carrying out comparative cross-cultural studies in different populations.

THE INTERNATIONAL PILOT STUDY OF SCHIZOPHRENIA (IPSS)

As underlined by Jablensky (1987), "Both the epidemiological and cross-cultural approaches to the study of schizophrenia have their birthdates around the turn of the century." Emil Kraepelin was one of the first psychiatrists to publish some cross-cultural observations on dementia praecox and manic-depressive illness after a trip to Java (Jablensky, 1989). Since then, other researchers have investigated the epidemiology and the clinical picture of schizophrenia in different cultures (Warner, 1985). However, it was only when WHO planned and started the IPSS that a comparative cross-cultural research on this disorder, carried out using a standardized reliable methodology, was made possible.

As shown in Table 1, the IPSS involved 9 centres in Africa, Asia, Europe and North America, with a total of 1,202 patients aged 15-44. The patients were selected for presence of psychotic symptoms and for absence of gross organic brain pathology, chronicity, alcohol- or drug-dependence, sensory defects and mental retardation. The majority of patients (811) had a clinical diagnosis of schizophrenia; the remaining 391 were classified as having affective disorders, reactive psychoses, neuroses, and personality disorders. Each patient has a detailed standardized clinical examination at the point of inclusion into the study and full reassessments two years later and five years later. The principal research instruments used in the IPSS were the Present State Examination, a psychiatric history schedule and a social description form.

TABLE 1. Summary of the WHO Studies on Schizophrenia

	INTERNATIONAL PILOT STUDY OF SCHIZOPHRENIA	WHO COLLABORATIVE STUDY ON PSYCHIATRIC DISABILITY	DETERMINANTS OF OUTCOME OF SEVERE MENTAL DISORDERS
NUMBER OF CENTRES	9	7	12
COUNTRIES	China (Taipei), Colombia, Czechoslovakia, Denmark, India, Nigeria, UK, USA, USSR	Bulgaria, Federal Republic of Germany, Netherlands, Sudan, Switzerland, Turkey, Yugoslavia	Colombia, Czechoslovakia, Denmark, India, Ireland, Japan, Nigeria, UK, USA, USSR
NUMBER OF PATIENTS	1,202	520	1,379
MAIN AREAS ASSESSED	Mental state (PSE), past history, social description, course and outcome	Mental state (PSE), past history, sociodemographic description, disability in social roles, behavioural impairments, pattern of course	Mental state (PSE), past history, course and outcome, disability in social roles, stressful life events, expressed emotion, perception of illness, family functioning
DIAGNOSIS	Clinical (ICD-8), computer (CATEGO), statistical clusters	Clinical (ICD-9), computer (CATEGO)	Clinical (ICD-9), computer (CATEGO), DSM-III (in some centres)
FOLLOW-UP	2 years, 5 years	1 year, 2 years, 5 years	1 year, 2 years

Source: Jablensky, 1987.

215

The main conclusions of the IPSS can be summarized in this way (WHO, 1979; Jablensky, 1984, 1987, 1989; Sartorius, 1988):

1. Schizophrenia is a universal disorder, which can be found both in the most industrialized areas of the world, and in developing countries and areas with a predominantly rural structure. Although in the IPSS no single symptom was invariably present in every patient and in every setting, the clinical pictures associated with a diagnosis of schizophrenia were remarkably similar at the level of symptom profiles. Patients diagnosed as schizophrenic tended to have high scores on lack of insight, suspiciousness, delusional mood, delusions or ideas of reference and persecution, flatness of affect, auditory hallucinations, and the delusion of being controlled by an external agency. Different proportions (between 31% and 85%, with an average of 56%) of the patients meeting the general criteria of a non-affective functional psychosis also exhibited one or more of the Schneider 'first-rank' symptoms, considered for many years as reliably distinguishing schizophrenia from other non-organic psychotic illnesses. These symptoms appeared to define a subpopulation of schizophrenia patients characterized by a generally high frequency and intensity of "positive" psychotic symptoms which manifested great similarity across the cultures.

2. Although schizophrenia is universal, there is great variability in terms of course and outcome. At the 2-year follow-up, which included 82% of the initial cohort, 37% of the patients were psychotic; 31% were symptomatic but not psychotic; and 32% were asymptomatic. On the whole, more than half of the patients were in the two groups with better prognoses.

3. Finally, the outcome at the 2-year follow-up and at the 5-year follow-up was significantly better for the patients from developing countries (Colombia, India, Nigeria) than for those from the other countries. This result was largely unexpected, but was confirmed even when it was controlled for certain variables, such as sex, age, and marital status. Out of all 9 countries, the two extremes of outcome were represented by strikingly different results in Nigeria and in Denmark. While in Nigeria about 57% of patients were in the group with the best outcome, in Denmark this number was only 6%. In a parallel manner, while in Nigeria only 5% of the patients were in the group with the worst outcome, in Denmark this group included 31% of the patients.

In the IPSS no single variable, and no combination of a few "key" variables, could explain much of the variation of any of the course and outcome measures in schizophrenia; in other words, no characteristics of the patient, of the environment, or of the initial manifestations of the disorder considered in isolation were an effective predictor of the subsequent course and outcome of the illness. The main variables associated with a positive outcome were an acute onset of the disorder, being married, a good work adaptation and the presence of affective symptoms. On the other hand a negative outcome was associated with a slow onset, being divorced or separated, being socially isolated, having received a prior psychiatric treatment, a long duration of the illness episode and a history of behavioural disorders.

The results of the 2-year follow-up have been amply confirmed at the 5-year follow-up, which included a total of 807 patients representing 76% of the initial cohort (Leff et al., 1990). Once again the patients from developing countries exhibited a clearly better outcome than the patients from developed countries. In terms of clinical outcome, measured by symptomatic status at time of follow-up, time spent in a psychotic episode and pattern of course, the Indian and Nigerian patients did much better than all the others. In addition, these patients and those from Colombia also showed an exceptionally good social outcome.

Figure 1 shows the different patterns of course at the 5-year follow-up (Sartorius et al., 1987). A significantly larger number of patients from developing countries had a course characterized by a single episode of illness, followed by full remission, or by many illness episodes, each followed by full remission. On the other hand, a significantly larger number of patients from developed countries showed either a course characterized by one or more episodes followed by incomplete remission, or a continuous condition of illness. All the different patterns of course correlated poorly with the initial diagnostic classification of the cases.

THE STUDY ON IMPAIRMENTS AND DISABILITIES IN SCHIZOPHRENIC PATIENTS

The second study aimed to explore the behavioural impairments and social disabilities in schizophrenic patients of recent illness onset. It included 520 patients in seven countries who were examined initially and also at one-year and two-year follow-up investigations (Table 1). In addition to the PSE and a history schedule, two new instruments, the WHO Disability Assessment Schedule (DAS) and the Psychological Impairments Assessment Schedule (PIRS), were developed for and used in this study. The PIRS was designed to describe and quantify negative symptoms, such as social and communication skills, while the purpose of the DAS was to elicit and rate data on social role performance and the environment factors influencing such performance.

The main results of this study can be summarized in this way (Jablensky, 1984, 1986, 1987):

1. There was a specific pattern in the occurrence of disabilities, in the sense that some social roles, with their behavioral correlates, were

FIGURE 1. Pattern of course in schizophrenia
5 year follow-up (IPSS)

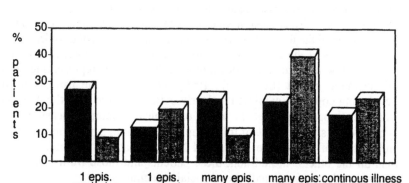

impaired before others; specifically, the area of sexual relationships tended to be impaired first, followed then by the work role. The area of self-care, which was initially preserved, became dysfunctional only when the majority of the other social roles had been impaired. In Table 2 the percentages of patients with dysfunctions in the main 7 social roles are shown: the range goes from a high of 74% of patients showing a dysfunction in sexual behaviour to a low of 35% of patients who exhibited a dysfunction in the area of self-care. This pattern could also be interpreted in the sense that a patient who exhibited a dysfunction in sexual behaviour, because this was the first area to be impaired, may not yet show disabilities in other areas, while a patient with a disability in the area of self-care was likely to already have a disability in the other areas.

2. Negative symptoms, such as inactivity, loss of interest and initiative, poverty of speech, etc., were the best predictors of outcome at the 5-year follow-up. Many similarities have emerged in patients from various centres in terms of frequency of diagnostically important syndromes, the nature and severity of psychological and behavioural impairments, and the pattern of development of social role dysfunctions.

THE STUDY ON THE "DETERMINANTS OF THE OUTCOME OF SEVERE MENTAL DISORDERS"

The third study, bearing the title "Determinants of the Outcome of Severe Mental Disorders," was undertaken in view of the great potential

TABLE 2. Number and Percentage of Patients with Social Role Dysfunctions, in up to 7 Roles, by Type of Social Role

ROLE	PATIENTS	
	n	%
Sexual relationship	198	74
Work role	171	64
Social withdrawal	158	59
Underactivity	156	58
Participation in household	138	52
Interests and information	136	51
Self-care	93	35
Total no. of patients	267	100

Source: Jablensky, 1986.

importance of the IPSS findings, and it focused more than the IPSS on the frequency of occurrence, the "natural history" of schizophrenia and the factors associated with differences in course and outcome. This study was based on more representative patient samples in different cultures (Sartorius et al., 1986). The case-finding strategy designed for the new study consisted of: (a) a prospective survey of specified psychiatric, other medical and social services in a given catchment area in each setting; and (b) identification of all individuals making a first lifetime contact with such services who exhibited signs and symptoms of a possible schizophrenic illness.

By extending the case-finding network to include a variety of "helping agencies" in the community (e.g., religious institutions, traditional healers), this strategy was expected to result in a better coverage of the incident cases of the disorder than the first inclusion method, although patients who never contacted any agency would still be missed.

Several research techniques which had earlier thrown light on specific facets of the course of schizophrenia were also used. These included the ascertainment of stressful life events prior to the onset of psychotic episodes, the measurement of expressed emotion in a key relative, the assessment of the perception of psychotic symptoms by the patient's family, and the evaluation of functional impairments and social disability. It was hoped that the application of these techniques would help to obtain data that could contribute to an explanation of the extraordinary finding of the IPSS that patients in developing countries on the whole have a better outcome than those living in developed countries.

The total population included in this second major study, which was carried out in 12 centres, 6 of which also participated in the IPSS, consisted of 1,379 subjects (745 men and 634 women) most of whom were urban residents (Table 1). With the exception of Ibadan, Cali and the rural area of Chandigarh, where most patients came from very poor neighbourhoods, the socio-economic status of the patients' neighbourhoods and households in the other centres was rated as "average" in comparison with local standards in the majority of cases.

The great majority (86%) of the 1,218 cases for which the beginning of the psychotic illness could be dated, had been identified by the case-finding network and assessed within 12 months of the onset of the disorder; in 61% of the cases this had occurred within 3 months.

The main results of this study can be summarized in this way (Jablensky, 1987, 1989; Sartorius, 1988; Sartorius et al., 1986, 1989):

1. Although there is a remarkable difference in incidence rates for schizophrenia diagnosed according to a broad definition, there is a striking similarity in incidence rates for schizophrenia diagnosed according to restrictive criteria. Adopting restrictive diagnostic criteria, the incidence of schizophrenia is more or less the same in all countries: 7-14 cases per year per 100,000 inhabitants aged 15-54 (Figure 2).

FIGURE 2. Incidence rates per 100,000
aged 15-54 (both sexes)

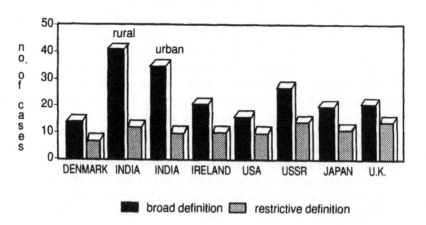

2. As already found in the IPSS, schizophrenic patients from developing countries have a course and an outcome significantly better than patients from developed countries. While 56% of the patients from developing countries exhibited a mild course, this percentage decreased to 39% for the patients from developed countries. Moreover, while only 24% of the patients from developing countries had a severe course, this percentage was 40% for the patients from developed countries. Regarding the type of onset, 36% of the patients under study had had an acute onset of the illness; the others had had a sub-acute or an insidious onset. However, as already found in the IPSS, the patients from developing countries had a greater frequency of acute onset (49%) compared to the patients from developed countries (26%), while the latter had more insidious onsets (43%) compared to the former (27%).

Figure 3 shows more specifically the differences between the patients on selected outcome variables; so, while 38% of the patients from developing countries were in full remission more than 3/4 of the follow-up time, compared to 22% of the patients from developed countries, only 16% of the patients from developing countries were on antipsychotic medication from 76% up to 100% of the follow-up time, compared to 61% of the patients from developed countries. While 55% of the patients from developing countries had never been hospitalized, this was true for only 8% of the patients from developed countries. Finally, while 15% of the patients

FIGURE 3. Differences between Patients on Selected Outcome Variables

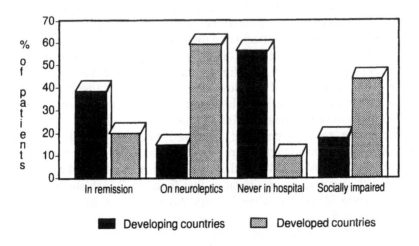

No. of patients studied: 1,014

from developing countries had impaired social functions throughout the follow-up time, 42% of the patients from developed countries were in this condition.

3. As shown in the IPSS, patients from developing countries showed a higher frequency of "voices speaking to the subject" and of visual hallucinations, while patients from developed countries showed more affective symptoms (mainly depressive) and a higher frequency of delusional mood and "thought insertion."

A high proportion of patients (from a low of 52% in Agra to a high of 92% in Prague) had made their first contact for the disorder under study with a health facility (psychiatric facility or GP); on the other hand 22% of patients in India and 31% of patients in Nigeria had made their first contact with an "alternative" facility (traditional healers or religious facilities). In 90% of the cases the reasons for contact were related to the occurrence or worsening of bizarre behaviour or of unintelligible speech, and to the deterioration of daily functions. In 26% of the cases it was possible to find a family member with a history of psychiatric disorders.

The most common sub-type of schizophrenia was paranoid schizophrenia (29% of the cases); in the developing countries about 10% of the patients were affected by catatonic schizophrenia.

As mentioned above, two sub-studies focused on the role of life-events and expressed emotion in the onset and course of schizophrenia.

In nine centres, among 386 patients studied with an acute onset, about 65% reported significant life events, independent from the illness, in the two or three weeks prior to the occurrence of the disorder (Day et al., 1987). Therefore it is confirmed that socioenvironmental stressors may precipitate schizophrenic attacks and that such events tend to cluster in the two to three week period immediately preceding illness onset. Interestingly, although the Indian and Nigerian centres reported many very acute onsets, they also reported very low rates of life events; therefore, on the basis of these results, the acute benign psychoses seen in these countries do not seem to be psychogenic (Bebbington, 1987).

Regarding schizophrenia and expressed emotion, patients from the Indian centre (Chandigarh) were compared to those from the Danish centre (Aarhus). While 54% of the Danish patients were rated as high on EE, which is a percentage similar to that found in British studies, in the Indian centre 30% of the urban families and only 8% of the rural families were classified as high EE. In particular, Indian relatives expressed significantly fewer critical comments, fewer positive remarks and less overinvolvement (Wig et al., 1987a, 1987b). The low proportion of high-EE relatives in the Indian sample was significantly associated with a low relapse rate (Leff et al., 1987).

CONCLUSIONS

What general conclusions can be drawn from this brief review of WHO studies on schizophrenia?

The first conclusion is that multicentric transcultural studies represent a valuable methodology for studying comparative psychiatric disorders and for understanding the influence which psychosocial and biological variables have on their pattern of course and outcome. They are feasible, and can also significantly improve research capabilities through the training of large groups of researchers and clinicians in the use of various research instruments. WHO is now planning a new long-term follow-up study, in which all patients included in the three studies discussed above, plus others included in a WHO study on dosage of neuroleptics in different populations, will be pooled in order to study the long-term course and outcome of the illness (O'Connor, 1990). This study will be the largest international long-term study on the course and outcome of schizophrenia ever undertaken and will include a total sample of more than 3,000 patients in 18 research centres. Data collection for this study would begin in June 1991 and would be completed within 12 months.

The second conclusion is that schizophrenia is universal, and patients with a diagnosis of schizophrenia in different populations and cultures share many features at the level of symptomatology. The incidence rates of the disorder are very similar across different countries and cultures. However, available evidence shows that socio-environmental factors play a very important role with regards to incidence, and also prevalence, of the disorder. Although the traditional social causation/social selection issue is still unresolved (Angermayer & Klusman, 1987; Dohrenwend et al., 1991), there are strong evidences which show a significant relationship between the socioeconomic status and the risk for schizophrenia. Data from the Epidemiological Catchment Area (ECA) Program shows that the estimated relative risk for schizophrenia in the lowest socioeconomic status groups was 7.85 (p < .001) compared to the highest socioeconomic status group and provides, according to the authors, "a quite dramatic confirmation of the findings reported by Hollingshead and Redlich a generation ago" (Holzer et al., 1986). Moreover Eaton (1985), in a review of the epidemiology of schizophrenia, concluded that the studies carried out show a consistent pattern in a using three basic categories of social class, it is common to observe a three-to-one difference in rates between the lowest and the highest class. Jablensky (1988), in a comprehensive review of the relationship between schizophrenia and the environment, stated that "Notwithstanding the methodological flaws of the early studies . . . , they have been consistent in finding a significant relationship between macrosocial variables and the epidemiology of schizophrenia." Also the finding of a substantial difference in the age of onset between males and females (Hafner et al., 1989) seems to confirm the importance of sociocultural factors in the occurrence of the disorder. In this context, it should be noted that a substantial decrease in the incidence of the disorder over the last few decades seems to have occurred, as shown in some specific studies (Munk-Jorgensen, 1986; Munk-Jorgensen & Jorgensen, 1986; Stromgren, 1986; Torrey, 1989; Sartorius et al., 1989; Beiser & Jacono, 1990; Der et al., 1990).

However, although universal, schizophrenia appears to have substantial variations in terms of course and outcome substantially different depending on the type of socio-cultural and socio-economic setting. Generally speaking, in the WHO studies the course and the outcome was significantly better for patients from developing countries than for those from developed countries, and this is confirmed by the results of many other studies (Warner, 1985). In addition, Warner (1985) has demonstrated that macrosocial variables, including the unemployment rate and the overall socioeconomic conditions of the society in which the patients live, can deeply affect the course and the outcome of schizophrenia, for instance in terms of recovery rates.

In any case, independent from the setting and contrary to the beliefs held in the psychiatric field for decades, there is a remarkable percentage of patients who recover from the illness. Table 3 shows the results of the major long-term follow-up studies of schizophrenia published between 1960 and 1991; in these studies, which were carried out over a follow-up period of up to 37 years, the percentage of patients clinically recovered ranged from a low of 6% to a high of 66%, with an average of 28% and a median value of 26%. The percentage of patients who showed a social recovery ranges from a low of 17% up to a high of 75%, with an average of 52% and a median value of 54%. Authors who have provided indepth reviews of the follow-up studies of schizophrenia have reached the same conclusion, stressing the possibility of social and/or clinical recovery for schizophrenic patients, even when institutionalized for decades (Harding, 1985; Warner, 1985; Ciompi, 1988, 1989; Wing, 1987; McGlashan, 1988; Shepherd et al., 1989; Wyatt et al., 1988). For this reason some authors have proposed a challenging view of the very concept of chronicity, stating that a variety of environmental and psychosocial factors can affect patient outcome and induce a misperception of chronicity (Ciompi, 1980; Harding et al., 1987).

It has been suggested that the existence of extended families may help to explain the better recovery rate for patients living in developing countries. To test this hypothesis, data from the 5-year and 10-year follow-up obtained within the IPSS at Cali, Colombia, have been compared with data from two 5- to 8-year follow-up studies of former schizophrenic inpatients of the Max Planck Institute of Psychiatry (MPIP) in Munich (Germany) (von Zerssen et al., 1990). Although schizophrenics in Cali are hospitalized and treated with drugs only during acute episodes of the psychosis and no facilities exist for long-term treatment, the psychopathological outcome was, on the whole, not worse than in Munich. Furthermore, the duration of hospitalization during the follow-up period was much lower in Cali compared to the German patients and a significantly lower number of Colombians were separated from their families. However, contrary to the hypothesis, family size did not predict course and outcome at both centers. The main results of the study concern the differences in the hospitalization rate and the degree of family integration during the course of the psychosis in an industrial and a developing country. They challenge the view that a highly developed professional care system is the best guarantee for improving the long-term course of schizophrenia. Rather, the integration of patients in a natural social environment, and the restriction of medical interventions to an indispensable degree may provide an optimal care strategy. This strategy is easier to realize in developing countries where the family structure is, on the whole, more intact than in industrialized countries with high divorce rates and a tendency to isolate the elderly and the sick from their families.

The third conclusion to be drawn from this review is that the results of the WHO studies are especially important when planning mental health services: according to their results, the vast majority of patients in developing countries and many patients in developed countries can be treated as out-patients, and in such circumstances their illness has a milder course.

The fourth and final conclusion is that some variables seem particularly important for predicting the general and long-term outcome of the illness. For instance, negative symptoms are especially important in this regard and should be given great importance when formulating treatment and rehabilitation plans. However, as underlined by Jablensky (1984), psychiatric services tend to pay much greater attention to the positive, often dramatic symptoms of psychosis, while they give less attention to the negative symptoms and to the impairments and dysfunctions in daily

TABLE 3. Clinical and Social Outcome in the Main Studies on the Long-Term Follow-up of Schizophrenia Published Between 1960-1991

AUTHOR, YEAR	COUNTRY	SELECTION YEARS	DURATION OF FOLLOW-UP (YEARS)	SIZE OF SAMPLE	FIRST ADMISSIONS (%)	MALE (%)	CLINICALLY RECOVERED (%)	POOR CLINICAL OUTCOME (%)	SOCIAL RECOVERY (%)
Affleck et al., 1976	U.K.	1959-61	12	155	?	51	?	24	48
Astrup et al., 1962	USA	1938-50	5-20	1102	100	53	20	63	59
Biehl et al., 1986	Germany	?	5	70	100	59	26	35	?
Bland & Orn, 1979	Canada	1963	14	90	100	?	21	37	65
Bleuler, 1978	Switzerland	1942-43	5-20	208	66	48	20	24	51
Brown et al., 1966	U.K.	1956	5	339	33	43	18	41	43
Ciompi, 1980	Switzerland	1963	mean 37	295	100	32	27	18	33
Gross & Huber, 1986	Germany	1945-59	21	502	-	-	26	35	56
Harding et al., 1987	USA	1955-60	20	82	0	50	-	40	60
Huber et al., 1975	Germany	1945-59	8-28	758	67	42	22	35	75
Kulhara & Wig, 1978	India	1966-67	5-6	174	100	?	29	32	72
Leon, 1989	Colombia	1968	10	84	-	-	43	25	50
Marinow, 1988	Bulgaria	?	20	280	-	-	-	27	51

McGlashan, 1984	USA	1950-75	15	163	0	52	6	41	--
Mignolli et al., 1991	Italy	1979	7	46	71	44	37	24	20
Munk-Jorgensen, 1989	Denmark	1972	13	53	100	-	23	50	24
Murphy & Raman, 1971	Mauritius	1956	12	113	100	?	59	36	71
Ogawa et al., 1987	Japan	1958-62	21-27	140	79	48	31	23	47
Salokangas, 1983	Finland	1965-67	7-8	175	100	47	26	24	69
Shepherd et al., 1989	U.K.	?	5	107	37	53	16	43	60
Stephens, 1970	USA	1948-59	5-16	472	100	?	23	28	?
Stone, 1986	USA	1963-76	10-23	94	-	-	8	-	-
Tsuang & Winokur, 1975	USA	1934-44	30-40	525	?	52	19	48	?
Vaillant, 1978	USA	1959-62	10	56	-	-	-	39	61
Verghese et al., 1989	India	1981-82	2	323	-	-	66	4	-
Watts, 1985	U.K.	1946-74	28	35	-	43	28	35	17
Waxler, 1979	Sri Lanka	1970-71	5-6	89	100	55	40	36	54
AVERAGE	--	--	14	243	86	48	28	32	52
MEDIAN VALUE	--	--	12	155	99	48	26	35	54

living of these patients. More attention given to the latter will result in an improvement in the therapeutic interventions.

In conclusion it is possible to agree with the statement expressed by Jablensky (1988): "The strongest evidence at present is that of an environmental effect on course and outcome of schizophrenia. Far from being an autochthonous, pre-programmed process, schizophrenia appears to be a dynamic development in which the quantity and quality of social stimuli, the emotional ambience of the family and the community, the demands of the society, and the ethos of treatment interact with the intrinsic neurophysiological vulnerability to shape the prognosis."

REFERENCES

Astrup, C., Fossum, A. & Holmboe, R. *Prognosis in Functional Psychoses,* Springfield: Thomas, 1962.

Bebbington, P., 'Life events and schizophrenia. The WHO collaborative study,' *Social Psychiatry, 22*:179-180, 1987.

Beiser, M. & Iacono, W.G. An update on the epidemiology of schizophrenia. *Canadian Journal of Psychiatry, 35*:657-668, 1990.

Biehl, H., Maurer, K, Schubart, C., Krumm, B. & Jung, E., 'Prediction of outcome and utilization of medical services in a prospective study of first onset schizophrenics: results of a five-year follow-up study,' *European Archives of Psychiatry and Neurological Sciences, 236*:139-47, 1986.

Bleuler, M. *The Schizophrenic Disorders: Long-Term Patient and Family Studies.* New Haven: Yale University Press, 1978.

Ciompi, L. Catamnestic long-term study on the course of life and aging of schizophrenics. *Schizophrenia Bulletin, 6*:606, 1980.

Ciompi, L., 'Learning from outcome studies,' *Schizophrenia Research, 1*:373-84, 1988.

Ciompi, L., 'Review of follow-up studies on long-term evolution and aging in schizophrenia,' in: *Schizophrenia and Aging,* New York: Guliford, 1989.

Day, R., Nielsen, A., Korten, A., Ernberg, G., Dube, K. C., Gebhart, J., Jablensky, A., Leon, C., Marsella, A., Olatawura, M., Sartorius, N., Stromgren, E., Takahashi, R., Wig, N. & Wynne, L.C., 'Stressful life events preceding the acute onset of schizophrenia: a cross-national study from the World Health Organization,' *Culture, Medicine and Psychiatry, 11*:123-205, 1987.

Der, G., Gupta, S. & Murray, R. Is schizophrenia disappearing? *Lancet, 335*:513-516, 1990.

Gross, G. & Huber, G., 'Classification and prognosis of schizophrenic disorders in light of the Bonn Follow-up Studies,' *Psychopathology, 19*:50-9, 1986.

Harding, C. M. & Strauss, J.S., 'The course of schizophrenia: an evolving concept,' in: Alpert, M. (ed.), *Controversies in Schizophrenia,* New York: Guilford, 1985, pp. 339-353.

Harding, C. M., Brooks, G. W., Ashikaga, T., Strauss, J. S. & Breier, A., 'The

Vermont Longitudinal Study of persons with severe mental illness, I: Methodology, study sample and overall status 32 years later,' *American Journal of Psychiatry, 144*:718-26, 1987.

Jablensky, A., 'Gli studi trans-culturali dell' Organizzazione Mondiale della Sanità' sulla schizofrenia: implicazioni pratich,' in: Faccincani, C., Fiorio, R., Mignolli, G. & Tansella, M. (eds.), *Le psicosi schizofreniche dalla ricerca alla pratica clinica,* Bologna: Patron, 1984, pp. 36-65.

Jablensky, A., 'Menomazioni e disabilità nei pazienti schizofrenici,' *Devianza ed Emarginazione, 11*:45-70, 1986.

Jablensky, A., 'Multicultural studies and the nature of schizophrenia: A review,' *Journal of the Royal Society of Medicine, 80*:162-67, 1987.

Jablensky, A., 'An overview of the World Health Organization multi-centre studies of schizophrenia,' 455-71. In: Williams, Paul & Rawnsley, K. (eds.), *The Scope of Epidemiological Psychiatry: Essays in Honour of Michael Shepherd,* London: Routledge, 1989, pp. 225-39.

Leff, J., Sartorius, N., Jablensky, A., Anker, M, Korten, A., Gulbinat, W. & Ernberg, G. The International Pilot Study of Schizophrenia. In: Hafner, H. & Gattaz, W.F. (eds.), *Search for the Causes of Schizophrenia,* Vol. II, Berlin: Springer, 1990, pp 57-66.

Leff, J., Wig, N.N., Ghoschizophrenia, A., Bedi, H., Menon, D. K, Kuipers, L., Korten, A., Ernberg, G., Day, R., Sartorius, N., & Jablensky, A., 'Expressed emotion and schizophrenia in North India, III: Influence of relatives' expressed emotion on the course of schizophrenia in Chandigarh,' *British Journal of Psychiatry, 151*:166-73, 1987.

León, C. A., 'Clinical course and outcome of schizophrenia in Cali, Colombia: A ten-year follow-up study,' *Journal of Nervous and Mental Disease, 177*:593-606, 1989.

Marinow, A., 'Prognosis and outcome in schizophrenia,' *International Journal of Mental Health, 17*:63-80, 1988.

McGlashan, T. H., 'The Chestnut Lodge Follow-up Study, II: Long term outcome of schizophrenia and the affective disorders,' *Archives of General Psychiatry, 41*:586-601, 1984.

McGlashan, T. H., 'A selective review of recent North American long-term follow-up studies of schizophrenia,' *Schizophrenia Bulletin, 14*:515-42, 1988.

Mignolli, G., Faccincani, C. & Platt, S., 'Psychopathology and social performance in a cohort of patients with schizophrenic psychoses. A 7-year follow-up study,' in: Tansella, M. (a cura di), 'Community-based psychiatry: long-term patterns of care in South-Verona,' *Psychological Medicine Monograph,* 1991 (in press).

Munk-Jorgensen, P., 'Why has the incidence of schizophrenia changed in Danish institutions since 1970?' *Acta Psychiatrica Scandinavica, 75*:62-8, 1987.

Munk-Jorgensen, P. & Mortensen, P. B., 'Schizophrenia: A 13-year follow-up,' *Acta Psychiatrica Scandinavica, 79*:391-9, 1989.

O'Connor, J. Largest international study on schizophrenia launched. *Psychiatric News, 25*:1, 16, 1990.

Ogawa, K., Miya, M., Watarai, A., Nakazawa, M., Yuasa, S. & Utena, H., 'A long-term follow-up study of schizophrenia in Japan–with special reference to the course of social adjustment,' *British Journal of Psychiatry, 151*:758-65, 1987.

Sartorius, N., 'Solving the conundrum of schizophrenia. WHO's contribution,' in: Stefanis, C. N. & Rabavilas, A. D. (eds.), *Schizophrenia. Recent Biosocial Developments,* New York: Human Sciences Press, 1988, pp. 23-38.

Sartorius, N., Jablensky, A., Ernberg, G., Leff, J., Korten, A. & Gulbinat, W., 'Course of schizophrenia in different countries: some results of a WHO International comparative 5-year follow-up study,' in: Hafner, H., Gattaz, W.F. & Janzarik, W. (eds.), *Search for the Causes of Schizophrenia,* Berlino: Springer, 1987, pp. 107-13.

Sartorius, N., Jablensky, A., Korten, A., Ernberg, G., Anker, M., Cooper, J. & Day, R., 'Early manifestations and first-contact incidence of schizophrenia in different cultures,' *Psychological Medicine, 16*:909-928, 1986.

Sartorius, N., Jablensky, A., Korten, A. & Ernberg, G., 'Course and outcome of schizophrenia: a preliminary communication,' in: Cooper, B. & Helgason, T. (eds.), *Epidemiology and the Prevention of Mental Disorders,* London: Rout-ledge, 1989, pp. 195-203.

Sartorius, N., Nielsen, J. A. & Strömgren, E. (eds.), 'Changes in Frequency of Mental Disorders over Time,' *Acta Psychiatrica Scandinavica Supplementum, 348*(79), 1989.

Shepherd, M., Watt, D., Falloon, I. & Smeeton, N., 'The natural history of schizo-phrenia: A five-year follow-up study of outcome and prediction in a represen-tative sample of schizophrenics,' *Psychological Medicine,* Monograph suppl. 15, 1989.

Stone, M. H., 'Exploratory psychotherapy in schizophrenia-spectrum patients,' *Bulletin of the Menninger Clinic, 50*:287-306, 1986.

Strömgren, E., 'Changes in the incidence of schizophrenia?' *British Journal of Psychiatry, 150*:1-7, 1987.

Torrey, E. F., 'Schizophrenia: Fixed incidence or fixed thinking?' *Psychological Medicine, 19*:285-87, 1989.

Tsuang, M. T. & Winokur, G. The Iowa 500: fieldwork in a 35-year follow-up of depression, mania and schizophrenia. *Canadian Psychiatric Association Jour-nal, 20*:359-365, 1975.

Vaillant, G. E. A 10-year follow-up of remitting schizophrenics. *Schizophrenia Bulletin, 4*:78-85, 1978.

Verghese, A., John, J. K, Rajkumar, S., Richard, J., Sethi, B. B. & Trivedi, J. K., 'Factors associated with the course and outcome of schizophrenia in India: Results of a two-year multicentre follow-up study,' *British Journal of Psychia-try, 154*:499-503, 1989.

Warner, R., *Recovery from Schizophrenia. Psychiatry and Political Economy,* London, Routledge, 1985.

Watts, C. A. H., 'A long-term follow-up of schizophrenic patients: 1946-1983,' *Journal of Clinical Psychiatry, 46*:210-6, 1985.

Wig, N. N., Menon, D. K., Bedi, H., Ghoschizophrenia, A., Kuipers, L., Leff, J.,

Korten, A., Day, R., Sartorius, N., Ernberg, G. & Jablensky, A., 'Expressed emotion and schizophrenia in North India, I: Cross-cultural transfer of ratings of relatives' expressed emotion,' *British Journal of Psychiatry, 151*:156-60, 1987.

Wig, N. N., Menon, D. K, Bedi, H., Leff, J., Kuipers, L., Ghosh, A., Day, R., Korten, A., Ernberg, G., Sartorius, N., & Jablensky, A., 'Expressed emotion and schizophrenia in North India, II: Distribution of expressed emotion components among relatives of schizophrenic patients in Aarhus and Chandigarh,' *British Journal of Psychiatry, 151*:160-65, 1987.

Wing, J. K, 'Has the outcome of schizophrenia changed?' *British Medical Bulletin, 43*:741-53, 1987.

Wyatt, R. J., Alexander, R. C., Egan, M. F. & Kirch, D. G., 'Schizophrenia, just the facts. What do we know, how well do we know it?' *Schizophrenia Research, 1*:3-18, 1988.

Zerssen, v. D., Leon, C. A., Moller, H. J., Wittchen, H. U., Pfister, H., Sartorius, N., 'Care strategies for schizophrenic patients in a transcultural comparison,' *Comprehensive Psychiatry, 31*:398-408, 1990.

ADDITIONAL REFERENCES

Angermayer, M. C. & Klusmann, D. (eds.), *From Social Class to Social Stress,* Berlin: Springer, 1987.

Dohrenwend, B. P., Levav, I., Shrout, P. E., Schwartz, S. B., Naveh, G., Link, B. G., Skodol, A. E., Steue, A., Socioeconomic status and psychiatric disorders: a test of the social causation-social selection issue, 1991 (in press).

Holzer, C. E., Shea, B. M., Swanson, J. W., Leaf, P. J., Myers, J. K., George, L., Weissman, M. & Bednarski, P., The increased risk for specific psychiatric disorders among persons of low socioeconomic status, *American Journal of Social Psychiatry, 6*:259-271, 1986.

Eaton, W. W., Epidemiology of schizophrenia, *Epidemiologic Reviews, 7*:105-126, 1985.

Jablensky, A., Schizophrenia and the environment, in: Henderson, S. & Burrows, G. (eds.), *Handbook of Social Psychiatry,* Amsterdam: Elsevier, 1988, pp. 8-116.

Hafner, H., Riecher, A., Maurer, K., Loffler, W., Munk-Jorgensen, P., & Stromgren, E., How does gender influence age at first hospitalization for schizophrenia? *Psychological Medicine, 19*:903-918, 1989.

Ciompi, L., Is chronic schizophrenia an artifact? Arguments and counter-arguments, *Fortshritte der Neurologie und Psychiatrie, 48*:237-248, 1980.

Harding, C. M., Zubin, J. & Strauss, J. S., Chronicity in schizophrenia: fact, partial fact or artifact? *Hospital and Community Psychiatry, 38*:477-486, 1987.

Steen, ..., Day, R., Sartorius, N., Emberg, G. & Anker, M. ... Cross-
emotion and schizophrenia in North India. A Cross-cultural transfer of culture
of relatives expressed emotion. *British Journal of Psychiatry* 147, 156-60,
1985.

Wahlberg, K.-E., Wynne, L. C., Oja, H., Keskitalo, P., Pykäläinen, L., Lahti, I.,
Moring, J., Naarala, M., Sorri, A., Seitamaa, M., Läksy, K., Kolassa, J.,
Tienari, P. Gene-environment interaction in vulnerability to schizophrenia:
findings from the Finnish Adoptive Family Study of Schizophrenia. *American
Journal of Psychiatry* 154, 355-362, 1997.

Wing, J. K. The concept of schizophrenia. *American Journal of Psychiatry*, 1981.

Wynne, R. J., Ventura, J., Luon, M. P. & Hardesty, J. P. ... Schizophrenia: the
role of stress. What do we know, how well do we know it? *Schizophrenia
Research* 14, 66, 1997.

Zubin, J., ..., Magaziner, D. & ..., ..., Steinhauer, S. R., ... A scientific
approach to diagnosis in schizophrenia: a neurobehavioral perspective. *Journal
of Abnormal Psychology* 99, 126-136, 1990.

ADDITIONAL REFERENCES

Aichhorn, M. E. & Klavetter, G. (eds.). *New Social Class*. New York,
Berlin: Springer, 1935.

Dohrenwend, B. P., Levav, I., Shrout, P. E., Schwartz, S. P., Naveh, G., Link,
B. G., Skodol, A. E., Stueve, A. Socioeconomic status and psychiatric disorders: a test of the social causation-social selection issue, 1992 (in press).

Halford, G. E., Shea, H. M., Cascardi, T. W., Lerer, R. J., Myers, A. K., Cooper, T.,
Weisman, M. M. Deinstitution, R. The decreased risk for specific psychiatric
disorders among divorce socioeconomic status. *American Journal of
Social Psychiatry* 62, 966-971, 1986.

Hahn, W. A. S. *Epidemiology of schizophrenia*. Rotterdam: ..., ..., 572-624,
1985.

Labowitz, A. Schizophrenia and the environment. In: Henderson, S. & Burrows, G.
(eds.). *Handbook of Psychiatry*. Amsterdam: Elsevier, 1984, pp. 51-70.

Mednick, A., Miezitis, A., Maurer, K., Loffler, W., Riecher-Rossler, P. & Suma-
gerl, T. How does gender influence age at first hospitalization for schizophrenia? *Psychological Medicine* 19, 903-918, 1989.

Mundt, C. ... Chronic schizophrenia: an artifact? Arguments and counter-arguments. *Fortschritte der Neurologie und Psychiatrie*, 48, 572-584, 1980.

Strömgren, G. M., Zubin, L. & Spring, I. S. Chronicity in schizophrenia: fact,
partial fact, or artifact? *Hospital and Community Psychiatry* 32, 977-986, 1981.